1.229

SOME TEXT HIGHLIG[

LAB £15

17/9779

A Text and Atlas of
Integrated Colposcopy

CHAPMAN & HALL MEDICAL ATLAS SERIES

Chapman & Hall's new series of highly illustrated books covers a broad spectrum of topics in clinical medicine and surgery. Each title is unique in that it deals with a specific subject in an authoritative and comprehensive manner.

All titles in the series are up to date and feature substantial amounts of top quality illustrative material, combining colour and black and white photographs and often specially-developed line artworks.

The amount of supporting text varies: where the illustrations are backed-up by large amounts of integrated text the volume has been called 'A text and atlas' to indicate that it can be used not only as a high quality colour reference source but also as a textbook.

A Text and Atlas of Integrated Colposcopy

For colposcopists, histopathologists and cytologists

M. C. Anderson, FRCPath, FRCOG
Senior Lecturer and Honorary Consultant
Previously at the Department of Histopathology
The Samaritan Hospital for Women, London, UK
Presently at the Department of Histopathology, University Hospital,
Queen's Medical Centre, Nottingham, UK

J. A. Jordan, MD, FRCOG
Consultant Gynaecologist
The Birmingham and Midland Hospital for Women, and
Birmingham Maternity Hospital, Queen Elizabeth Medical Centre,
Birmingham, UK

A. R. Morse, CFIAC
Principal Cytologist
Department of Cytology and Experimental Pathology, St Mary's
Hospital Medical School, and The Samaritan Hospital for Women,
London, UK

F. Sharp, MD, FRCOG
Professor of Obstetrics and Gynaecology
The University of Sheffield, Northern General Hospital,
Sheffield, UK

CHAPMAN & HALL MEDICAL
London · New York · Tokyo · Melbourne · Madras

UK	Chapman & Hall, 2–6 Boundary Row, London SE1 8HN
JAPAN	Chapman & Hall Japan, Thomson Publishing Japan, Hirakawacho Nemoto Building, 7F, 1-7-11 Hirakawa-cho, Chiyoda-ku, Tokyo 102
AUSTRALIA	Chapman & Hall Australia, Thomas Nelson Australia, 102 Dodds Street, South Melbourne, Victoria 3205
INDIA	Chapman & Hall India, R. Seshadri, 32 Second Main Road, CIT East, Madras 600 035

First edition 1992

© 1992 Chapman & Hall

Designed by Thin Blue Line
Typeset in 10/12pt Palatino by Opus Design

Printed in Hong Kong by
Thomas Nelson (Hong Kong) Ltd

ISBN 0 412 38490 6

British Library Cataloguing in Publication Data

A text and atlas of integrated colposcopy: For
  colposcopists, histopathologists and cytologists.
  1. Women. Uterus. Cervix. Diagnosis. Colposcopy
  I. Anderson, M.
  618.1407545

ISBN 0–412–38490–6

Contents

Preface

We have been organizing and teaching on colposcopy courses for many years, and this book is an attempt to put together all the information that we would like to impart on the courses if the time were available.

This volume is primarily intended for colposcopists, therefore the bulk of it covers the colposcopic appearances of the cervix in health and disease, largely in the form of an atlas. However, the book is much more than an atlas of colposcopy, as the colposcopist needs to be familiar with the factors responsible for the causation of disease and its histogenesis, as well as with the histological and cytological means of diagnosis which necessarily complement the colposcopic approach. The sections on histology and cytology have been incorporated in such a way that they will also be of value to the histologist and cytologist working alongside the colposcopist.

In addition to the basic 'core' chapters on histology, cytology, colposcopic appearances and treatment of disease of the cervix, vagina and vulva, we have also included chapters discussing policies of referral for colposcopy, setting up a colposcopy service, and training considerations. These wider issues are particularly important to everyone involved with colposcopy.

Although our book contains elements of an atlas and a textbook, it covers more ground than either of these could. By adopting this wider approach, we believe that we have satisfied a need for a book that provides in one volume all the information required by colposcopists and those working with them.

Malcolm C. Anderson, *Nottingham*
Joseph A. Jordan, *Birmingham*
Anne R. Morse, *London*
Frank Sharp, *Sheffield*

January 1991

Foreword

This excellent working text and atlas, written by four experts in the fields of colposcopy, histology and cytology, is timely in its appearance.

The authors have worked closely together over many years, on numerous courses given at the Royal College of Obstetricians and Gynaecologists, as well as nationally and internationally. This book is a distillation of the knowledge and expertise gained in their own clinical work and enhanced by their very extensive teaching experience. The authors are all international experts in their own right.

The text is authoritative and clear in its meaning, the complementary skills and value of cytology, histology and colposcopy are emphasized, and the excellent illustrations greatly enhance the written word.

Having had the privilege of collaborating with all four authors over the years in various capacities, and working closely with Mrs Anne Morse and Dr Malcolm Anderson over the past twenty years, it is a special honour for me to 'cap' those ties by writing the foreword for a book which deserves, and I believe will achieve, international acclaim.

George Pinker
Consultant Gynaecologist, St Mary's Hospital and The Samaritan Hospital for Women, London

1. The Normal Cervix

NORMAL STRUCTURE

General features

The uterus is composed of the upper, muscular body and the lower, more fibrous cervix; the 'internal cervical os' marks the junction between the two. Approximately one half of the cervix protrudes into the vaginal vault through its anterior wall, and the other half remains supravaginal. The part of the cervix lying in the vagina is referred to as the 'portio vaginalis', or often merely as the 'portio'.

The cervix varies considerably in size and shape, depending on age and parity, but it is typically cylindrical, about 3 cm in length and 2.5 cm in diameter.

The 'external os' is an imprecise landmark, marking the point at which the cervical canal opens out into the vagina.

The 'cervical canal' connects the uterine cavity with the vaginal lumen, extending from the external to the internal os, and is flattened from front to back.

Tissue lying outside the external os is described as 'ectocervical', and inside the canal as 'endocervical'. Histopathologists tend to use the terms 'ectocervical' and 'endocervical' in a descriptive manner, to indicate original squamous or glandular tissue respectively, without taking into account its anatomical position on the cervix. This may give rise to confusion; for example, a biopsy taken from the vaginal surface of the cervix may be reported as showing endocervical tissue, where eversion has occurred. The colposcopist should be aware of this frequent, but permissible, looseness of terminology.

Epithelial covering

Epithelium covering the cervix is initially of two types: squamous and columnar. It is laid down during embryological development, and is referred to as 'original' or 'native' epithelium.

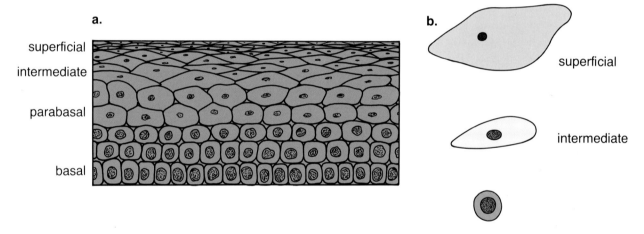

a.

superficial
intermediate
parabasal
basal

b.

superficial

intermediate

Fig. 1.1 Diagrammatic representation of (a) the histology of original cervical squamous epithelium, and (b) the cytology of normal squamous cells.

Fig. 1.2 Original squamous epithelium. H&E, × 32.

Fig. 1.3 Original squamous epithelium. Basal and parabasal layers are seen. H&E, × 128.

SQUAMOUS EPITHELIUM
Histological appearances
The original squamous epithelium covers the ecto-cervix and is continuous with the vaginal epithelium. It is stratified, non-keratinizing epithelium, which is separated from the underlying stroma by a slightly undulating basal lamina.

In describing both normal and abnormal squamous epithelium, the terms 'differentiation', 'maturation' and 'stratification' are frequently used. These terms are closely interrelated in meaning, but are not quite synonymous.

Differentiation
Differentiation refers to the process in which the squamous cell becomes fully functional as a flattened, protective layer. In the skin, full differentiation involves keratinization, but in the normal cervix differentiation falls short of this. In normal epithelium, maturation and differentiation are virtually synonymous, i.e. the cells differentiate as they mature.

In abnormal epithelium, in common with other premalignant and malignant states, the term 'differentiation' relates to the degree of morphological and functional similarity between abnormal and normal cells at all stages of maturation. Therefore, the equivalence of 'differentiation' with 'maturation' diminishes as the epithelium becomes more abnormal.

Maturation
Maturation is very closely related to differentiation in meaning, and characterizes the changes seen in cells as the surface of normal squamous epithelium is reached. A mature squamous cell must also show good differentiation, but an immature squamous cell may show some degree of differentiation that enables it to be recognized as squamous in type.

Stratification
Stratification is a necessary consequence of maturation and differentiation; it refers to the way in which the epithelium is divided into layers of progressively more mature and flattened cells as the surface is reached.

The processes of differentiation, maturation and stratification are illustrated in Fig. 1.1. The maturing squamous epithelium of the ectocervix has a well defined basal layer attached to the basal lamina (Figs 1.2 and 1.3). These cells have a large nuclear cytoplasmic ratio. The parabasal cells form the next few layers, and these also have a high nuclear cytoplasmic ratio with rather basophilic cytoplasm. It is in this layer that occasional mitotic figures are normally seen.

Further maturation and differentiation (Fig. 1.4) produces the intermediate cells in which the cyto-plasm is more abundant, often with a prominent space containing glycogen around the nucleus (Fig. 1.5). These cells often form a 'basket weave' pattern (see Fig. 1.2). The cytoplasm becomes more abundant as maturation progresses, and the nucleus becomes smaller, so that cells in the intermediate zone are slightly flattened with round nuclei of moderate size, in which the chromatin pattern is readily discernible.

The intercellular 'prickles' are usually very promi-nent in the skin and characterize the stratum spin-osum of normal skin. Although these are a diagnostic feature of squamous cell carcinoma, they are not so striking in the cervical epithelium, but may be identified in the parabasal and, with more difficulty, in the intermediate layer. Further maturation of the squamous cells produces the superficial layer of epithelium (see Fig. 1.4). This layer is composed of

Fig. 1.4 Original squamous epithelium. Intermediate and superficial cells are seen. H&E, × 128.

Fig. 1.5 Original squamous epithelium. This has been stained to demonstrate glycogen. Periodic acid Schiff, × 32.

3

markedly flattened cells, with eosinophilic cytoplasm and small, slightly flattened nuclei. At this final stage of maturation the nuclei become pyknotic, small and very dense, with no nuclear structure discernible within them.

The fully mature and differentiated cell of the squamous epithelium is very flat, and its nature is probably better appreciated when the cell is seen lying flat in a cytological preparation, rather than when cut across in a histological section.

Cytological features

The cytological features of normal squamous cells closely reflect the histological appearances (Fig. 1.6). However, the overall size of the cell and size of the nucleus, together with the differential staining of the cytoplasm, are of paramount importance to the

Fig. 1.6 A normal cervical smear appearance, with a mixture of superficial and intermediate squamous cells. A small sheet of endocervical glandular cells can be seen at the centre. Papanicolaou stain, × 128.

cytologist. Thus, the type of stain used, as well as the subtle variations associated with it at cellular level, are of great relevance.

The standard method for staining cytological preparations is that of Papanicolaou. Haematoxylin is used to stain the nucleus of cells blue/black. Other counterstains (EA50 and OG6) will stain the cytoplasm various hues of green to blue and pink, depending on the maturity of differentiation of the cell as a result of changes in cell metabolism and chemical reactions in the cytoplasm.

Throughout this book, all references to cytological staining and the colours observed at microscopy relate to the use of Papanicolaou stain.

Parabasal squamous cells

Parabasal squamous cells have a large nucleus which occupies approximately 80–90% of the overall cell size. The nucleus is darkly stained, with a well defined, coarse chromatin pattern. The cytoplasm has a thick, homogeneous appearance, and stains green or blue. The cell has a rounded shape, with well defined cell borders (see Fig. 1.6).

Intermediate squamous cells

As the cell matures, the amount of cytoplasm increases in relation to cell size and also to nuclear cytoplasmic ratio. The cytoplasm retains an affinity to basophilic staining but becomes 'thinner' and more transparent, characteristically staining pale blue. It may show a well defined region around the nucleus, which stains yellow; this denotes the presence of glycogen.

The nucleus of the intermediate squamous cell is

Fig. 1.7 Atrophic pattern. The smear consists of regularly sized parabasal cells, many of which have shed their cytoplasm and consist of bare nuclei. Papanicolaou stain, × 128.

Fig. 1.8 Prolapse. The original squamous epithelium is showing hyperkeratosis with a prominent granular layer. H&E, × 32.

4

round, with an obvious chromatin structure; however, this is pale stained and finely granular, not showing the hyperchromasia and coarseness associated with the parabasal cell.

Superficial squamous cells
As maturation progresses, squamous cells from the superficial layers of the epithelium become larger, with a pink staining, almost transparent cytoplasm. The cells are flattened, with angled edges suggesting a polyhedral shape. The nuclei are very small and dense, with no visible chromatin structure, and are referred to as pyknotic.

Keratinization is not a normal occurrence in the cervix, and maturation of normal squamous epithelial cells is arrested at this point. However, when genital prolapse occurs, keratinization may be seen on a section, along with some thickening of the epithelium (Fig. 1.7). The keratinized superficial cells are often readily recognized with cytology (Fig. 1.8).

Hormonal response
The squamous epithelium of the cervix is responsive to hormonal stimuli, and is dependent on oestrogen for full development. If oestrogen is deficient, or its effects are counteracted by high levels of progesterone, full maturation does not take place and cells at the surface of the epithelium do not become fully differentiated.

Following the menopause, the cells do not mature beyond the parabasal stage. As a result, the epithelium becomes atrophic, i.e. thin and composed of cells that have a relatively high nuclear cytoplasmic ratio, with virtually no flattening as the surface is reached (Fig. 1.9). Glycogen is absent, as maturation does not reach the intermediate cell stage. A rather similar appearance is seen during the late stages of pregnancy, and even more markedly in the postpartum period.

The cyclical changes are best observed in vaginal smears, but they are also seen in normal cervical smears. The most striking change is an alteration of the ratio of superficial to intermediate squamous cells during the normal menstrual cycle. These basic changes can be measured by the karyopyknotic index (KPI): this represents the percentage of superficial squamous cells with pyknotic nuclei, to intermediate cells (parabasal cells are excluded), based on a minimum count of 200 cells.

Oestrogen effect/proliferation
Following menstruation, the proportion of superficial squamous to intermediate squamous cells rises towards midcycle; the smear is dominated by superficial squamous cells, although a few intermediate cells are still seen (normal range KPI: 80–90%). At this time, the cells are nicely displayed in flat sheets, with a clean background and few polymorphs (Fig. 1.10).

Secretory changes and progesterone effect
After ovulation, the effect of oestrogen suppression by progesterone is reflected in the increasing proportion of intermediate to superficial cell types. At this time, cells tend to clump together in large clusters, with poorly differentiated cell borders or folded and curled edges (Fig. 1.11). There is an increase in background debris and polymorphs

Fig. 1.9 Prolapse. The atrophic pattern is usually retained, with parabasal cells predominating. Random superficial squamous cells are present, which sometimes show marked keratinization. Papanicolaou stain, × 128.

Fig. 1.10 Postmenopausal squamous epithelium. H&E, × 128

(Fig. 1.12), which may make a cellular assessment difficult, if not impossible, and also unreliable.

Menstrual appearances
A smear taken during menstruation consists mainly of red blood cells, with small groups of darkly staining endometrial cells (Figs 1.13 and 1.14). Predictably, the squamous cell detail is often obscured, making the specimen unacceptable for a reliable assessment. The optimal time for taking a smear is midcycle. Therefore, if possible, arrangements for smear tests should be made with this in mind.

Postmenopausal atrophic pattern
In the postmenopausal woman, the cervical smear pattern is composed almost entirely of parabasal and low intermediate cell types, with no cyclical changes and rarely any endocervical glandular cells (see Fig. 1.7).

A similar pattern may be seen postpartum, although the presence of squamous metaplasia, endocervical glandular cells and regenerative changes are frequently noted, making possible a distinction from atrophy of the postmenopausal type.

Fig. 1.11 Superficial squamous cells at midcycle. A fully developed oestrogen effect is seen with a clean background. Papanicolaou stain, × 128.

Fig. 1.12 Day 19 of the menstrual cycle. The intermediate cells are showing clumping and folding, with occasional glycogenated cells. Some polymorphonuclear leucocytes are present. Papanicolaou stain, × 128.

Fig. 1.13 Day 24 of the menstrual cycle. Clumping and folding of the cells are more pronounced features. There are numerous polymorphonuclear leucocytes and cell debris in the background. The appearance is untidy, and can often render the smear unsatisfactory for assessment. Papanicolaou stain, × 128.

Fig. 1.14 Menstrual pattern. Small groups of comparatively darkly stained endometrial cells in a bloodstained background. This appearance often makes a reliable cytological assessment impossible. Papanicolaou stain, × 128.

COLUMNAR EPITHELIUM

Histological appearances
Architectural features
The caudal limit of the field of endocervical epithelium is the original squamocolumnar junction. At its cephalic extreme, the endocervical epithelium merges (through a zone of isthmic endometrium, several millimetres in length) with endometrial epithelium of the lower part of the uterine body. The columnar epithelium of endocervix lines the cervical canal, forms crypts that pass deep into the substance of the cervix, and develops into papillary projections protruding into the lumen of the canal.

Endocervical crypts may extend as far as 1 cm from the surface of the cervix, but usually they are much more superficial (Fig. 1.15). Although often loosely termed 'glands', their structure is not that of a true gland in that there is no duct leading to acini. Endocervical crypts are elongated, branching tunnels, and are lined by the same epithelium which lines the canal on the surface.

The endocervical epithelium is not a simple, flattened surface, and particularly in the few millimetres immediately above the squamocolumnar junction it forms multiple papillary projections. Colposcopically, these 'grape-like' villi are the hallmark of endocervical tissue (see Chapter 7). Each villus is covered by a single layer of columnar epithelium, and has a core of superficial endocervical stroma containing a single vessel (Fig. 1.16).

Cellular features
In the normal, unaltered state, the endocervical epithelium is a single layer of tall, columnar cells with regular basal nuclei, giving a 'picket fence' appearance (Fig. 1.17). The cytoplasm contains finely dispersed mucin (Fig. 1.18). Goblet cells are not characteristic of endocervical epithelium. Some ciliated cells are normally present.

Not uncommonly, areas of tubal metaplasia are seen in the endocervical crypts. Developmentally, this may well be heterotopia rather than metaplasia, and care must be taken not to confuse its appearance with that of glandular atypia. Epithelium of endometrial type may sometimes also be seen in the

Fig. 1.15 Endocervical crypts. H&E, × 12.8.

Fig. 1.16 Endocervical villi. H&E, × 32.

Fig. 1.17 Original columnar epithelium. H&E, × 128.

Fig. 1.18 Original columnar epithelium. This has been stained to show mucin. Alcian Blue, × 128.

cervix. (These features are discussed in greater detail in Chapter 11.)

Cytological features

Glandular cells of endocervical origin are loosely referred to by cytologists as endocervical cells (Figs 1.19, 1.20). In general, these cells are easily identified, particularly since they frequently occur in small groups and sheets, although occasionally whole villi may be seen (Fig. 1.21).

The nuclei are basophilic and darkly stained with a prominent but finely granular chromatin structure, sometimes with chromocentres or small nucleoli. The nuclei are basally located in a cylindrically shaped cell. The cytoplasm stains a rather pale blue/grey (although occasionally pink hues can be seen), and is finely vacuolated with poorly defined cell borders.

Endocervical cells are approximately five times the size of lymphocytes, and somewhat smaller than mature squamous cells. When seen end-on, they appear round with a small rim of pale blue/grey cytoplasm. A differential diagnosis between para-basal and endocervical cells may be difficult.

CERVICAL POLYPS

Cervical polyps are extremely common, and consist of a localized overgrowth of endocervical tissue. Most are symptomless, but sometimes they present with irregular vaginal bleeding.

The polyp is composed of the lamina propria of the endocervix, with surface epithelium and underlying crypts. The surface epithelium may be ulcerated, and the underlying tissue may then take on the features of granulation tissue; this is often seen with symptomatic polyps. When the surface epithelium is present, it very often shows squamous metaplasia of varying degrees of maturity. Moreover, the superficial stroma is commonly infiltrated by inflammatory cells, with plasma cells being predominant among them.

Associated with squamous metaplasia, a polyp is frequently found to contain dilated endocervical crypts. Sometimes it may be composed solely of a few mucus-filled cysts covered by a layer of metaplastic squamous epithelium.

Endocervical polyps must be distinguished from polyps arising in the endometrium, and also from

Fig. 1.19 Endocervical glandular cells. These are showing palisading with a typically columnar shape and basally located nuclei. The cytoplasm is finely vacuolated. Papanicolaou stain, × 128.

Fig. 1.20 A nicely displayed clump of endocervical cells. The typical 'honeycomb' appearance of the cells is seen when viewed end-on. Some cells at the edge of the group are of a characteristic, cylindrical shape. Papanicolaou stain, × 128.

Fig. 1.21 Endocervical villus. Cytologically, this is seen as a darkly stained, dense cluster of cells. The columnar cells on the surface can be seen at higher magnification, but the core of the villus is composed of stromal cells. Papanicolaou stain, × 128.

fibroid polyps, both of which may extend into the endocervical canal and protrude through the external os. It must also be remembered that cervical intraepithelial neoplasia can affect the surface epithelium of a polyp, usually in association with this condition involving another area of the transformation zone. However, sometimes the polyp may bear the only recognizable cervical intraepithelial neoplasia.

Stroma

The stroma of the cervix is fibromuscular. Layers nearest to the surface are predominantly composed of rather loose fibrous tissue, with muscle lying deeper, beyond the field of the more superficial crypts (Figs 1.22 and 1.23). Muscular tissue is more superficial beneath the ectocervical squamous epithelium than in the endocervix.

Several small blood vessels are present in the cervical stroma, forming a subepithelial plexus beneath the columnar epithelium. Those, together with the vessels within the endocervical villi, contribute to the formation of characteristic abnormal vascular patterns of mosaic and punctation (for the colposcopic appearances see pages 83 and 84).

The superficial cervical stroma almost invariably contains an infiltrate of inflammatory cells, usually plasma cells and lymphocytes, particularly in the region of the squamocolumnar junction (Fig. 1.24). Unless extreme, this infiltrate should not be considered pathological; it represents the response to a continuous low grade stimulation by a variety of antigenic factors.

TRANSFORMATION ZONE

Squamocolumnar junction

Ideally, the squamocolumnar junction would be situated at the external os (Fig. 1.25), so that squamous epithelium lies on the ectocervix and columnar epithelium lines the canal. This seems to be what the two types of epithelium are best suited for. However, in the great majority of women this is not the encountered configuration; it is this deviation from the 'ideal' anatomy of the cervix that is the starting point of a chain of events which may eventually lead to invasive squamous cell carcinoma.

Fig. 1.22 Endocervix showing stroma. The deep, denser, muscular layer is seen at the bottom of the field. H&E, × 12.8.

Fig. 1.23 Endocervical stroma. Typical spindle cells are seen. H&E, × 128.

Fig. 1.24 Squamocolumnar junction. This shows a sparse, chronic inflammatory infiltrate in the superficial stroma. H&E, × 12.8.

Hormonal changes

At the time of puberty and during adolescence, the female genital tract enlarges in response to increasing levels of ovarian hormones and continuing stimulation by the physiological levels that are soon reached. This increase in size is most apparent in the body of the uterus, but the cervix also enlarges and alters in shape; the most significant element of this alteration is an eversion which appears to be concomitant with a 'rolling out' of the ectocervical component (this process is illustrated by comparing Figs 1.25 and 1.26).

Development of the transformation zone

The process of eversion causes a change in the position of cervical epithelium, so that epithelium initially lining the lower part of the cervical canal is now situated on the vaginal portion of the cervix (see Fig. 1.26). When viewed with a vaginal speculum, a red area is seen to surround the external cervical os, corresponding to the area of everted endocervical tissue. The term 'erosion' has traditionally been applied to this appearance; at first, this may not seem an inappropriate term, as the tissue shows redness and roughness at naked eye examination, suggesting that it is ulcerated and haemorrhagic.

Redness is due to the more vascular endocervical stroma seen through the thinner 'filter' of endocervical epithelium, and roughness is a consequence of the villous nature of everted endocervical epi-

thelium. Therefore, erosion is a term that is best not used, as it implies an erroneous view of the phenomenon.

A variety of alternative terms have been used, such as 'erythroplakia', 'ectopy' and 'transformation zone'. It is in this zone that physiological transformation to metaplastic squamous epithelium takes place (Fig. 1.27).

More importantly, this is the area where transformation to cervical intraepithelial neoplasia occurs, which may lead to invasive squamous cell carcinoma of the cervix. In fact, this area should not be called 'a transformation zone' until squamous metaplasia has started to develop. The transformation zone is defined as the area of cervix bounded caudally by the original squamocolumnar junction, and cephalically by the highest point that squamous metaplasia reaches.

The transformation zone may be described as normal, either immature or mature, abnormal, or congenital. These concepts will be discussed in separate sections.

Other hormonal effects on the squamocolumnar junction

Apart from adolescence, eversion of the cervix occurs at other times, although it is thought that this period is by far the most significant in the development of cervical malignancy. In the neonatal period, the effect of maternal hormones on the fetus leads to eversion of the cervix. In pregnancy, increased levels of

Prepubertal Cervix

columnar endocervical epithelium and crypts

original squamo-columnar junction

original squamous epithelium

Fig. 1.25 'Ideal' cervix. The squamocolumnar junction is situated at the external cervical os. The arrows show the direction of the movement which takes place as a result of the increase in bulk of the cervix during adolescence.

Postadolescent Cervix (a)

original squamo-columnar junction

Fig. 1.26 Process of eversion. On completion, endocervical columnar tissue lies on the vaginal surface of the cervix, and is exposed to the vaginal environment.

circulating hormones cause the cervix to evert further, beyond the position reached at the end of adolescence. After each pregnancy, the cervix will return to more or less the state that it was in before that pregnancy. The combined oral contraceptive pill has a similar but less marked effect on the degree of eversion.

After the menopause, the levels of sex steroid hormones fall and the eversion reverses (Fig. 1.28) so that the transformation zone passes back into the cervical canal. The original squamocolumnar junction may come to lie further within the canal than it did in childhood. This process of inversion may commence as many as ten years before the menopause, and for this reason the whole of the transformation zone may be visible at colposcopy in older women.

Squamous metaplasia

CONCEPT AND STIMULI

As described above, eversion leaves endocervical epithelium on the vaginal portion of the cervix. This epithelium is highly differentiated and specialized, performing its function most effectively within the cervical canal. The vaginal environment is hostile to this delicate epithelium, as the most important difference between the endocervical and vaginal environments is the much higher acidity in the vagina of a woman of reproductive age, which has been found to be even more marked in pregnancy. This feature is most significant in stimulating the epithelium to undergo squamous metaplasia, whereby an area initially covered by columnar epithelium becomes covered by squamous epithelium.

Mature, fully differentiated epithelial cells cannot change into another type of epithelial cell; the process is one of replacement, in which columnar cells are lost and replaced, not by more columnar cells as would normally happen in the endocervix, but by cells that will eventually differentiate into mature squamous cells.

This process of squamous metaplasia on the cervix is physiological and should be considered a normal event. There is nothing sinister about it, and its relationship with squamous cell carcinoma of the cervix is only that the two conditions share the same early path in the process of their development.

RESERVE CELL HYPERPLASIA

The first sign that the process of squamous metaplasia is beginning in the endocervix is the appearance of reserve cell proliferation. Reserve cells are seen as a single layer of cells beneath and very close to the nuclei of columnar epithelial cells, initially giving the impression that the epithelium has a double line of nuclei.

The origin of reserve cells is not clear; it seems likely that they are normally present in small numbers beneath the endocervical columnar epithelium, and replenish the cells as they are lost.

Alternative but less probable origins may be the endocervical stromal cells and blood-borne mono-

Postadolescent Cervix (b)

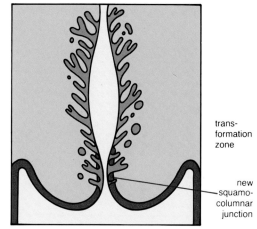

new squamo-columnar junction

trans-formation zone

Postmenopausal Cervix

trans-formation zone

new squamo-columnar junction

Fig. 1.27 Postadolescent cervix. Acidity of the vaginal environment is one of the factors which encourage squamous metaplastic change, replacing the exposed columnar epithelium with squamous epithelium.

Fig. 1.28 Postmenopausal cervix. At this time, cervical eversion, which was so important in adolescence, reverses; thus, the transformation zone is now drawn into the cervical canal. The original squamocolumnar junction may be situated further within the canal than it was before puberty (see Fig. 1.25), and the new squamocolumnar junction may be out of sight, high inside the canal.

cytes. Morphologically, reserve cells have a somewhat similar appearance to the basal cells of the original squamous epithelium, with round nuclei and little cytoplasm. As the metaplastic process continues, reserve cells proliferate and form a layer which is several cells thick. At this stage, the endocervical villi begin to fuse; this development can be appreciated both histologically (Fig. 1.29) and colposcopically (see Chapter 7).

It has also been suggested that the basement membrane of the original columnar epithelium dissolves as reserve cells appear, and is reformed between the proliferative reserve cells and the stroma, as metaplasia continues.

Cytologically, reserve cells appear as small, round cells with a very darkly staining nucleus and coarsely textured chromatin in a small amount of green staining cytoplasm (Fig. 1.30). When they occur discretely, they may well be overlooked or be mis-taken for lymphocytes or endometrial cells. However, reserve cells are most frequently seen with columnar endocervical cells.

IMMATURE METAPLASIA

As the metaplastic process develops further, reserve cells begin to undergo differentiation and maturation, to become initially immature squamous cells. The amount of cytoplasm increases a little, and the nuclei enlarge, often with prominent nucleoli.

Stratification of the epithelium is not apparent at this stage. Residual groups of mucin-containing columnar cells may often be seen both on the surface of immature squamous epithelium and embedded within it (Fig. 1.31); this may be subsequently described as showing immature and incomplete squamous metaplasia. At this stage the epithelium is usually thin, and the junction between epithelium

Fig. 1.29 Reserve cell hyperplasia. H&E, × 128.

Fig. 1.30 Reserve cell hyperplasia. Small, darkly stained cells with large nuclei and a small rim of cytoplasm are seen. Papanicolaou stain, × 128.

Fig. 1.31 Immature, incomplete squamous metaplasia. H&E, × 128.

Fig. 1.32 Immature squamous metaplasia. As reserve cells become more mature metaplastic cells, the nucleus is less prominent, although still showing its chromatin structure. The outline of the cell is elongated and resembles more closely that of a squamous cell. Papanicolaou stain, × 128.

and stroma often presents a 'scalloped' outline, reflecting the fact that endocervical villi have been fused together by the process of immature squamous metaplasia.

For the cytologist, the most important aspect in recognizing metaplastic cells in cervical smears is an appreciation of the spectrum of cell changes that invariably occur, and an awareness that cells of varying degrees of maturation will be seen in any single cervical smear.

In cytology, the term 'immature' is used to describe cells which have a round shape, with a thick, green staining cytoplasm and a very large, darkly staining nucleus showing a coarse chromatin pattern, sometimes with prominent chromocentres or small nucleoli. Occasionally, the cytoplasm may show some elongation, and the cell tends to take on an oval shape (Fig. 1.32).

Fig. 1.33 Mature squamous metaplasia. Note the opening of a crypt. H&E, × 32.

Fig. 1.34 Maturing squamous metaplasia. This shows the features that distinguish a metaplastic cell from a mature squamous cell. The nucleus is now much smaller than that of an immature metaplastic cell, and the cytoplasm closely resembles the shape and texture of a squamous cell. Papanicolaou stain, × 128.

MATURE METAPLASIA

As the process of squamous metaplasia continues, the developing squamous cells become more mature. Eventually, the epithelium has fully mature, differentiated squamous cells on its surface, and no residual columnar cells are seen. It is now of almost the same thickness as the original squamous epithelium (Fig. 1.33), and is glycogenated. The purpose of the metaplastic process is fulfilled when the delicate, thin layer of endocervical, columnar cells is replaced by a much thicker, stronger and more protective layer of squamous cells.

As maturation of the metaplastic process progresses, the cytoplasm appears more squamous in nature, staining blue or pink, but not quite achieving the characteristic, transparent appearance of the normal, intermediate cell. The cytoplasm gradually becomes more recognizably squamous, taking on a pink hue; the nucleus becomes less dominant, with a less obvious chromatin structure, although it still appears larger in comparison to the nucleus of a normal squamous cell (Fig. 1.34).

In complete maturity, the metaplastic cell is cytologically indistinguishable from the normal superficial squamous cell that arises from the original squamous epithelium.

METAPLASIA AND CRYPTS

Although squamous metaplasia is most often seen as a process of the surface epithelium, it may involve the crypts of the endocervix, albeit usually only the more superficial ones (Fig. 1.35). The pattern of this involvement can become quite complex, and the inexperienced pathologist must be wary of misinter-

Fig. 1.35 Squamous metaplasia, involving gland crypts. H&E, × 12.8.

preting these appearances as invasive carcinoma. This misdiagnosis may be avoided by looking at the cell detail of both the overlying epithelium and the apparent invasive islands.

NATURAL HISTORY OF METAPLASIA

In the cervix, squamous metaplasia is an irreversible process: columnar epithelium that has been replaced by squamous epithelium cannot revert to columnar again. Thus, when the transformation zone recedes into the cervical canal after the menopause (see Fig. 1.28), the epithelium remains squamous. It also seems likely that once the process of transformation has started, the stimulus must be maintained if the process is to continue and be completed. However, it is not always true that the process of squamous metaplasia, once started, progresses rapidly and inexorably to completion. If the stimulus is withdrawn, for instance, by a reversed cervical eversion or reduced acidity of the upper vagina, the metaplastic process may be arrested at any stage. Equally, if the stimulus recurs, progression towards a mature squamous epithelium may recommence.

Furthermore, squamous metaplasia may progress at varying rates in different areas of the same cervix, perhaps reflecting a range of degrees of protection that the cervical mucus offers the epithelium. It is, therefore, very common to observe areas of widely differing maturity in the metaplastic squamous epithelium within the transformation zone.

CONGENITAL TRANSFORMATION ZONE

Histological appearances

The congenital transformation zone (CTZ) is confusing to pathologists as well as to colposcopists. It is poorly understood and not always recognized. The condition is not at all rare, and has been seen in approximately 5% of all women examined at the Colposcopy Clinic of the Samaritan Hospital, London.

The congenital transformation zone is a variant of squamous metaplasia, and has many histological features in common with the latter. Maturation of the squamous epithelium is not fully completed, and typically the congenital transformation zone shows a disorder of maturation which combines excessive maturation on the surface, as exemplified by keratinization, with delayed, incomplete maturation of the deeper layers. These deeper layers show the same features as squamous metaplasia; the nuclei are large but regular, with prominent nucleoli. There is

little pleomorphism, and mitotic figures are infrequent. Rapid maturation may occur within the course of the thickness of three or four cells.

Hyperkeratosis or parakeratosis (layers of keratinized cells with retained, although pyknotic, nuclei) is very often present on the epithelial surface. When this layer is thick, it corresponds to leucoplakia which is one of the characteristic colposcopic features of the congenital transformation zone (see Chapter 7).

The most striking histological feature of the congenital transformation zone is the irregularity of the lower margin, the epithelial/stromal junction, which is always dentate, with apparent incursions of squamous epithelium into the stroma (Fig. 1.36). Very often, the tips of these processes appear to be separated from the overlying epithelium, giving the impression of invasive buds. This impression may be further heightened when the centre of the process undergoes differentiation, so that a whorl of keratin is seen in the centre (Fig. 1.37). Careful attention to the cytological details of the section will show that the congenital transformation zone is not an invasive neoplasm.

Cytologically, cells arising from an area of congenital transformation zone will, in general, be indistinguishable from cells arising from the typical transformation zone. However, personal observation (ARM) has led to a belief that, occasionally, cells from an area of immature congenital transformation zone may show exaggerated nuclear features, with very coarsely clumped and densely stained chromatin. Therefore, a differential diagnosis between immature metaplastic cells and cervical intraepithelial neoplasia may be difficult.

V. SUPERFICIAL cf crypts deep

Fig. 1.36 Congenital transformation zone. Normal, original squamous epithelium is present on the left. H&E, × 12.8.

HISTOGENESIS

The colposcopic and histological appearance of the congenital transformation zone are the same as some of those seen in diethylstilboestrol exposure in utero (see Chapter 19), and it is possible that the mechanism of development of both conditions is similar in some respects.

During embryogenesis, the cuboidal epithelium of the canalized vaginal anlage is replaced by squamous epithelium, a process that is thought to start at the caudal end of the urogenital sinus. This process would normally reach completion, so that the entire length of the vagina and ectocervix becomes covered by squamous epithelium well before the time of birth. If, however, the upward conversion of cuboidal to squamous epithelium happens to be arrested, then some cuboidal epithelium will remain. This epithelium may undergo squamous conversion later in intrauterine life, and perhaps even after birth. The line of demarcation between congenital transformation zone and original squamous epithelium is the point at which normal squamous development stopped, and therefore the congenital transformation zone is believed to be the result of this delayed squamous change.

The difficulty with this theory of histogenesis is that it does not justify the spiky lower margin of the epithelium, which can only be explained as a replacement of superficial gland crypts by metaplastic cells of the congenital transformation zone, but remnants of these gland crypts are not seen. More work is needed to elucidate fully the origin of the congenital transformation zone.

NATURAL HISTORY OF THE CONGENITAL TRANSFORMATION ZONE

The morphological appearances of the congenital transformation zone through the microscope suggest that it is more closely related to squamous metaplasia than to cervical intraepithelial neoplasia, although the colposcopic features have much in common with the latter (see Chapter 7). However, observation of women with areas of untreated congenital transformation zone has shown no propensity to malignant change over several years of follow up. The finding of a diploid chromosome content by microdensitometry provides further support for the suggestion that the condition has no malignant potential. Gradual maturation of the epithelium is expected over the years, with increased glycogenation.

Fig. 1.37 Congenital transformation zone. Keratinization is seen in the centre of one of the 'pegs'. H&E, × 32.

15

2. Cervical Intraepithelial Neoplasia

NOMENCLATURE

For many years, the premalignant changes of the cervical epithelium were known as the dysplasias and carcinoma in situ (CIS). The definitions of these abnormalities were not precise, and left much to the interpreter. Carcinoma in situ was defined as 'a lesion in which all or most of the epithelium shows the cellular features of carcinoma', whereas dysplasia was 'all other disturbances of differentiation of squamous epithelium, of lesser degree than carcinoma in situ'.

The chief disadvantage of the dual dysplasia/CIS terminology was that it suggested a distinction between the dysplasias, which were often considered to be benign epithelial changes, and carcinoma in situ, the name of which implied significant malignant potential, if not actual malignancy.

These imprecise definitions allowed histopathologists to exercise considerable flexibility in interpreting epithelial changes. For instance, epithelium showing differentiation and stratification (suggesting a diagnosis of dysplasia) may also show a marked degree of nuclear abnormality, leading to its wrong allocation to the category of carcinoma in situ.

This looseness of interpretation worsened the imprecision and subjectivity in reporting cervical epithelial abnormalities. When this approach by pathologists was superimposed on a clinical approach, whereby carcinoma in situ was sometimes overtreated and dysplasia was in some cases inadequately treated, it became apparent that a rather unsatisfactory situation existed which allowed the vague histological concepts of the disease to be compounded by imprecise clinical management protocols.

Over the last three decades, it has become clear that the range of intraepithelial abnormalities of the cervix belong to one disease process, the components of which vary in degree. 'Cervical intraepithelial neoplasia' (CIN) was suggested as the term appropriate to this spectrum of disease, and it is now being increasingly used. However, practitioners have to be familiar with both systems of nomenclature, as occasionally the dysplasia/carcinoma in situ terminology is still used.

The concept of cervical intraepithelial neoplasia proposes that all degrees of abnormality should be given the same name, as part of a continuous spectrum of disease, so that the mildest form of cervical intraepithelial neoplasia is equivalent to mild dysplasia, and the most abnormal forms are the same as carcinoma in situ (Table 2.1). CIN 3 includes both severe dysplasia and carcinoma in situ; this point is important in that it recognizes the lack of actual

Table 2.1 Correlation between cervical intraepithelial neoplasia and dysplasia/carcinoma in situ

CIN 1	CIN 2	CIN 3	
Mild dysplasia	Moderate dysplasia	Severe dysplasia	Carcinoma in situ

difference between severe dysplasia and carcinoma in situ, which relieves the histopathologist of the problem of distinguishing between them.

The arguments in favour of the 'cervical intraepithelial neoplasia' terminology are (Table 2.2):
1. The unitary terminology is in accord with the modern management approach, whereby cervical intraepithelial neoplasia is regarded as one disease.
2. It is more readily reconcilable with what is known of the nature and natural history of the disease.
3. It recognizes that some of the mildest forms of cervical intraepithelial neoplasia constitute one end of the spectrum which may lead to invasive carcinoma, so that they may be dealt with accordingly.

On the other hand, critics of the 'cervical intraepithelial neoplasia' terminology have claimed that the labelling of very minor, often reversible, and perhaps reactive changes as neoplastic, increases the chances of dealing with them too radically. An understanding of the histopathology of the conditions concerned, together with an appreciation of the guidelines for treatment laid out in this book, should minimize this difficulty.

HISTOLOGY

Diagnosis

The histopathologist has to make the decision whether or not the epithelium in a cervical biopsy shows cervical intraepithelial neoplasia and, if so, its degree. The histological features which are used to establish the diagnosis are listed in Table 2.3.

STRATIFICATION, DIFFERENTIATION AND MATURATION

The meaning of each of these closely related terms has been discussed in Chapter 1. Two aspects are taken into account when assessing a case of cervical intraepithelial neoplasia. First, it should be readily apparent whether or not there is any maturation and stratification. This used to be the main criterion for

Table 2.2 Cytological and histological terminology

	Normal		CIN 1	CIN 2	CIN 3	
Histological diagnosis	Other benign conditions	Squamous metaplasia	Mild dysplasia	Moderate dysplasia	Severe dysplasia	Carcinoma in situ
Preferred cytological diagnosis	Normal/ Inflammatory changes	Squamous metaplasia	Mild dyskaryosis	Moderate dyskaryosis	Severe dyskaryosis	
Alternative cytological diagnosis	Normal/ Inflammatory atypia	Squamous metaplasia	Dyskaryosis		Malignant cells	
Papanicolaou class	Class 1 + 2		Class 3	Class 4	Class 5	
Department of Health class	Class 2		Class 3	Not classified	Class 4	
Vague diagnosis	Normal		Atypical			

distinguishing carcinoma in situ from severe dysplasia: if no maturation was seen, then the lesion was carcinoma in situ, whereas the presence of differentiation indicated a diagnosis of severe dysplasia, a distinction which currently does not seem relevant.

Secondly, the proportion of thickness of epithelium showing maturation and differentiation can be used as a measure of severity in a case of cervical intraepithelial neoplasia. If epithelial cells begin to differentiate, with associated maturation and resultant stratification in the basal quarter of the epithelium, the degree of abnormality is likely to be less severe than where this change is not apparent until the superficial quarter of the epithelium is reached.

In other words, the more severe degrees of cervical intraepithelial neoplasia are likely to have a greater proportion of the thickness of epithelium composed of undifferentiated cells, with only a narrow or nonexistent layer of mature, differentiated cells on the surface. However, this is only one of a number of relevant criteria, and should not be taken as the sole criterion, or indeed as the most important one.

Table 2.3 Histological features of CIN

1 **Differentiation, maturation, stratification**
   a) Present or absent
   b) Proportion of the thickness of epithelium showing differentiation

2 **Nuclear abnormalities**
   a) Increased nuclear cytoplasmic ratio
   b) Hyperchromasia
   c) Nuclear pleomorphism
   d) Anisokaryosis

3 **Mitotic activity**
   a) Number of mitotic figures
   b) Height in epithelium
   c) Abnormal configurations

NUCLEAR ABNORMALITIES

These are the familiar cytological features which are applied in the diagnosis of dyskaryosis in cervical smears. Increased nuclear cytoplasmic ratio, hyperchromasia, nuclear pleomorphism and variation in nuclear size (anisokaryosis) are all very important features to be taken into account when abnormal epithelium is being assessed.

Enlargement and irregularity of the nuclei are related to the chromosomal abnormalities that have so often been described in cervical intraepithelial neoplasia, although it would seem hazardous to attempt to distinguish between aneuploidy and polyploidy in ordinary histological preparations.

Fig. 2.1 CIN 2. This is an unusual appearance, as the nuclear changes in the basal three or four layers of cells are quite marked. On the other hand, maturation is well developed and less than one-third of the epithelium is showing severe abnormalities. An argument could be made for designating this a CIN 3, on the basis of the abnormalities of the basal layers. H&E, × 128.

In general terms, there is good correlation between the proportion of epithelium showing maturation and the degree of nuclear abnormality. However, when there is lack of correlation, the degree of nuclear abnormality should be taken as the more reliable criterion in grading.

A comparison of Figs 2.1 and 2.2 illustrates this dilemma: Fig. 2.1 shows an epithelium which is beginning to mature in its middle third, but the nuclei of the basal third show marked abnormalities. Conversely, Fig. 2.2 illustrates an example where maturation is not seen until the top third of the epithelium is reached, but nuclear atypia is quite mild. The former is the more abnormal epithelium, even though the latter has a greater thickness of undifferentiated cells; both have been designated CIN 2.

MITOTIC ACTIVITY

Mitotic figures are present in normal squamous epithelium of the cervix, but they are infrequent and are seen only in the parabasal layers. In cervical intraepithelial neoplasia, the number of mitotic figures increases, and these may be seen not only in the parabasal zone but also higher up in the epithelium. The height in the epithelium at which mitotic figures are found is generally much the same as the level reached by immature cells; the less differentiation in an epithelium, the higher the level at which mitotic figures are likely to be seen.

This is expected, as both mitotic activity and lack of differentiation are expressions of immaturity of cells. At this point, it should be noted that infection with human papillomavirus can produce several morphological changes in the epithelium (see Chapter 12). One of these changes is an increase in

Fig. 2.2 CIN 2. Mitotic figures are quite frequent, and one is seen in the upper half of the epithelium. Nevertheless, the uniformity of nuclei and good maturation justify calling this lesion CIN 2 rather than CIN 3. H&E, × 32.

Fig. 2.3 Abnormal mitotic figure; three-group metaphase. The mitotic figure on the left has most of its chromatin at the equatorial plane, but two smaller clumps are present at either end and have not migrated. The mitotic figure on the right is normal. H&E, × 128.

the number of mitotic figures, which may result in attributing an erroneously high grade to a cervical intraepithelial neoplasia.

In addition to the number of mitotic figures and their height in the epithelium, note is also taken of abnormal configurations of mitotic figures. The most common aberration is the three-group metaphase (Fig. 2.3), which is seen when most of the chromosomes line up along the equatorial plane of the cell at metaphase, but small collections of chromosomes are left at the poles of the cells. If mitosis is completed, these non-moving elements will confer an uneven distribution of chromatin to the daughter cells. This could be a mechanism by which aneuploidy is perpetuated in an abnormal epithelium. Less

common than the three-group metaphase are mitotic figures with more than two spindles, such as the triaster (Fig. 2.4) and quadraster mitotic figures. Other rare forms may also be encountered.

Keratinization

Keratinization may be seen on the surface of cervical intraepithelial neoplasia. It is most frequently found in CIN 3 (Fig. 2.5), but may also sometimes occur with minor forms of cervical intraepithelial neoplasia, the congenital transformation zone and even otherwise normal metaplastic epithelium.

Colposcopically, keratinized epithelium will be seen as leucoplakia; it should be borne in mind that an invasive carcinoma may be hidden under an area of leucoplakia.

GRADING OF CERVICAL INTRAEPITHELIAL NEOPLASIA

Grading may be characterized as follows, taking into account the histological features described above.

CIN 1

There is usually good maturation. Nuclear abnormalities are present, although of minimal degree. These are mainly confined to the deeper layers of the epithelium, but some nuclear abnormalities persist at the surface; if this were not so, cytological recognition of CIN 1 would not be possible. Mitotic figures are present, but not numerous, and do not show abnormal configurations (Fig. 2.6).

Fig. 2.4 Abnormal tripolar mitotic figure. Three spindles have formed, instead of the normal two. H&E, × 128.

Fig. 2.5 Keratosis on CIN 3. This thick layer of keratin is very obvious colposcopically as leucoplakia. The granular layer is also prominent (see Fig. 8.7, page 85). H&E, × 32.

Fig. 2.6 CIN 1. Slight nuclear abnormalities with little pleomorphism and hyperchromasia are seen. Enlarged nuclei persist to the surface, and maturation is obvious. H&E, × 128.

CIN 2

Maturation is present in the upper half of the epithelium, again with some nuclear atypia persisting at the surface. Nuclear abnormalities are more marked and extend higher in the epithelium than those of CIN 1 (Fig. 2.7). Abnormal mitotic figures may be seen, and these may be present throughout the basal half of the epithelium (Figs 2.8 and 2.9; see also Figs 2.1 and 2.2).

CIN 3

Differentiation and stratification may be completely absent, or present only in the superficial quarter of the epithelium. Nuclear abnormalities may extend through the entire thickness of the epithelium, and are more marked in degree than in CIN 1 and CIN 2 (Fig. 2.10). Mitotic figures may be numerous, and abnormal forms are frequent (Figs 2.11–2.16).

Fig. 2.7 CIN 2. Nuclear crowding is moderate in the basal part of the epithelium. Cytoplasm increases in amount as the surface is reached. A few cells show koilocytotic change. H&E, × 128.

Fig. 2.8 CIN 1–2. Nuclear pleomorphism is apparent, and a mitotic figure is seen halfway up the epithelium. There is abundant cytoplasm in most cells, and maturation is good. As cervical intraepithelial neoplasia is a spectrum, it is quite legitimate to refer to intermediate forms, such as CIN 1–2 or CIN 2–3. H&E, × 128.

Fig. 2.9 CIN 2–3. Mitotic figures are numerous, two being seen halfway up the epithelium. Very good maturation is present on the surface. H&E, × 128.

Fig. 2.10 CIN 3. On the right side of the field, there is marked nuclear enlargement with crowding and one giant nucleus. There is some surface maturation. The maturation is better on the left, and some of the more superficial cells show koilocytotic change. H&E, × 128.

Fig. 2.12 CIN 3. Many mitotic figures are distributed throughout the thickness of the epithelium. H&E, × 128.

Fig. 2.11 CIN 3. A fairly thin epithelium, showing almost full thickness loss of differentiation. Mitotic figures are very prominent, several being abnormal. Even so, most cells have a fair amount of cytoplasm. H&E, × 128.

Fig. 2.13 CIN 3. Stratification is seen in one to four or five layers of cells. Nuclear abnormalities are striking. H&E, × 128.

Fig. 2.14 CIN 3. There is virtually no surface maturation or stratification. Mitotic figures are sparse. H&E, × 128.

Fig. 2.15 CIN 3. A particularly thick example, up to 40 cells thick in places. H&E, × 32.

Fig. 2.16 CIN 3. In contrast to Fig. 2.15, this is a remarkably thin epithelium, but the nuclear pleomorphism and hyperchromasia justify the diagnosis of CIN 3. H&E, × 128.

Subjectivity of diagnosis

The diagnosis and grading of cervical intraepithelial neoplasia are made on a combination of apparently distinct, but often interrelated, morphological criteria. Many of these are features that vary in degree, in quantitative terms, but not in a way that can be precisely measured; their interpretation, therefore, is largely subjective and a matter of opinion.

Furthermore, these criteria have to be applied with different priority to different examples of cervical intraepithelial neoplasia: one example may show numerous mitotic figures, with many abnormal forms but little nuclear abnormality. Another example may show few mitotic figures, but striking nuclear pleomorphism and hyperchromasia. Both are examples of CIN 3, but in each one the morphological criteria have to be applied in slightly different ways.

This introduces further subjectivity into the histological interpretation of cervical intraepithelial neoplasia, so much so that a lesion described by one pathologist as CIN 1 may be diagnosed by another as CIN 3. To make matters worse, it has been demonstrated that even the same pathologist may interpret a slide of cervical intraepithelial neoplasia differently on separate occasions.

These inconsistencies further support the concept of cervical intraepithelial neoplasia as one disease, which is irreconcilable with subdivisions, and the allocation of grades is fraught with exactly the same difficulties that were encountered with the dysplasia/carcinoma in situ terminology.

CRYPT INVOLVEMENT

Cervical intraepithelial neoplasia develops in the transformation zone, the field of columnar epithelium that undergoes squamous metaplasia. It follows the contours of the original columnar epithelium, and affects gland crypts as well as the surface.

Gland crypt involvement by cervical intraepithelial neoplasia is often recognizable at colposcopy, and is usually obvious in histological sections (Figs 2.17 and 2.18). In a study of 354 cone biopsies of women with CIN 3, it was found that 88.6% had some degree of crypt involvement. The mean depth of crypt involvement was 1.24 mm, and the mean plus 3 standard deviations (99.7% of the population under study) was 3.8 mm. The latter figure is the depth of tissue that must be consistently and effectively removed for adequate treatment of cervical intraepithelial neoplasia by any method.

Other studies have shown that the depth of crypt involvement increases as cervical intraepithelial neoplasia becomes more severe, as does the size of the area affected by it.

Diagnosis

It is important that crypt involvement is correctly diagnosed and not misinterpreted as invasive carcinoma. Features that help the histopathologist to recognize crypt involvement and distinguish it from invasion are as follows:

1. Crypt involvement occurs in the area where the crypts are found, so that normal or partially

Fig. 2.17 Crypt involvement by cervical intraepithelial neoplasia. This is a mounted section from a cone biopsy. Very extensive crypt involvement is present; there is no invasion. The dilated crypt is lined by CIN 3 and, at its deepest point, this cervical intraepithelial neoplasia is just over 6 mm from the surface epithelium in the canal. × 1.

Fig. 2.18 Crypt involvement by cervical intraepithelial neoplasia. The crypt occupying the centre of the field has been cut off-centre, resulting in a non-apparent lumen. Because all the cells are fairly close to the basement membrane, there may be an impression that this epithelial abnormality is more severe than it really is. H&E, × 32.

affected crypts are often seen alongside crypts in which the columnar epithelium is entirely replaced by cervical intraepithelial neoplasia (see Fig. 2.17).

2. Involved crypts have a smooth outline and are surrounded by a basement membrane. Around them, the stroma may show some circumferential thickening of the fibrous tissue.

3. Cells of cervical intraepithelial neoplasia occupying the crypts have the same morphological appearances as cells of the overlying epithelium. This feature may not be obvious if the crypt is cut off-centre, or if the intraepithelial neoplasia completely fills the crypt; in this case, the abnormal epithelium does not have a surface, so maturation appears to be less than that on the surface (see Fig. 2.18).

On the other hand, invasive carcinoma, particularly in the early stages, is frequently composed of cells which are better differentiated than those of the intraepithelial neoplasia from which it arises (a finding which is discussed in detail in Chapter 10). Thus, a focus of cells with more abundant, eosinophilic cytoplasm, is a useful clue to the possibility of invasion.

4. The stroma surrounding a focus of microinvasion often shows a reaction to the infiltrating tumour. There may be an increase in the content of lymphocytes locally, or loosening of the stroma; often, both features are seen together. The stroma around areas of crypt involvement by cervical intraepithelial neoplasia is similar to that under the neoplasia at the surface; if lymphocytes are present, as they very frequently are beneath the neoplasia, then the infiltrate is fairly uniform, and not focused on one or two particular points.

Attention to these points helps to distinguish between crypt involvement by cervical intraepithelial neoplasia and early invasion. However, even to the experienced pathologist this distinction remains a constant problem. Oblique cuts of involved crypts can be very difficult indeed to distinguish from invasion (Fig. 2.19).

Further difficulty is caused by the fact that invasion may sometimes take place by means of rounded islands of infiltrating carcinoma, apparently surrounded by basement membrane.

EXFOLIATIVE CYTOLOGY

The confusing and controversial situation concerning the nomenclature of intraepithelial abnormalities, coupled with varying opinions of interpretation among histopathologists, as discussed above, can create difficulties in cytological classification and interpretation.

Cytology is the vital link between clinician and patient; it is the initial indication that all is not well, and that further investigation may be necessary. The clinician, therefore, relies on the cytologist to give an assessment which is as accurate as possible of the type and degree of abnormality, in a clear and concise report. This will enable the clinician to decide on the course of management, and to advise the patient accordingly. Reassurance and a repeat smear after a specified interval may be all that is necessary, or a more thorough explanation and referral for colposcopy with a view to treatment may be indicated.

Cytological reporting

Various forms of reporting are used, and some of these are shown in Table 2.2.

Most cytologists are aware that a descriptive report using unequivocal terms, together with a recommendation regarding further management, is the type of report most acceptable to clinicians, whether in specialist gynaecological clinics, family planning clinics or general practice. This strategy has been recently recommended by the British Society for Clinical Cytology Working Party on Terminology in Gynaecological Cytology (Table 2.4). A vague report will convey nothing of real value to the clinician, thus rendering further investigation mandatory, albeit quite unnecessarily in many instances.

Although the 'cervical intraepithelial neoplasia'

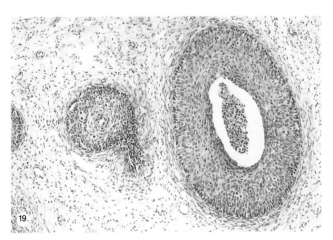

Fig. 2.19 Crypt involvement by cervical intraepithelial neoplasia. The smaller of these two crypts appears to have a spiky projection arising from it, giving the impression of early invasion. However, there is no stromal reaction at this point, and the cells have not changed in morphological appearance. This is an oblique cut of a smaller branch of the crypt. H&E, × 32.

Table 2.4 BSCC terminology guidelines

1 Unsatisfactory for assessment (state reason)
2 Negative
3 Nuclear changes bordering on mild dyskaryosis
4 Dyskaryotic cells: mild
                        moderate
                        severe
5 Malignant cells suggestive of invasive
   carcinoma: squamous cell
                        adenocarcinoma

Table 2.5 Cytological features of dyskaryosis

Nuclear changes
Enlargement
Variation in size and shape
Hyperchromasia
Abnormal appearance and distribution of chromatin
Irregular nuclear outline
Irregular thickening of nuclear membrane
Nucleoli
Mitoses

Cytoplasm
Variable
Indication of degree of dyskaryosis

terminology is used by histopathologists, it is inappropriate for a cytological approach, since cytological criteria must be based on individual cell changes rather than whole tissue patterns that cervical intraepithelial neoplasia refers to. The term 'dyskaryosis' is, therefore, preferred. For convenience, and to align it as closely as possible with the histological grades, thus facilitating a coherent approach, dyskaryosis is arbitrarily subdivided into mild, moderate and severe degrees. These three grades correlate to the histological grades of CIN 1, CIN 2 and CIN 3 respectively.

The advent of colposcopy, with the resultant availability of histological material from CIN 1 and CIN 2, has enabled the cytologist to compare cytological appearances with histological patterns to an extent that was previously not possible. The cone biopsy was for many years the only treatment for intraepithelial abnormalities, and this procedure was not frequently undertaken until the cellular changes indicated a severe lesion. Although it would be wrong to suggest that cytology should be used to diagnose the precise degree of cervical intraepithelial neoplasia, it is often possible for an experienced cytologist to assess a particular degree with accuracy.

It is important that cytologists exercise some discrimination between the grades of dyskaryosis, as in Britain colposcopy clinics are still expanding to cope with the number of women with abnormal smears who need to be selectively referred, at least initially, for colposcopy.

It is also vital that cytologists understand the nature of an unsatisfactory smear and the importance of reporting it as such, rather than as 'negative' or, worse still, 'showing vague inflammatory change or "irregular" features' (see page 48). These reports do not assist in the management of patients, they erode clinical confidence in the cytologist, and may result in leaving a malignancy unrecognized.

CYTOLOGICAL FEATURES

The cytologist relies heavily on individual cell changes for recognizing dyskaryosis and differentiating between degrees of dyskaryosis, in contrast to the histopathologist, who examines the features of the whole tissue and relationships between cells, in addition to cellular detail.

The way that cells are distributed in a cervical smear may bear little relationship to their relative positions in situ. However, it is a well established fact that changes in the cells from the uppermost layers of epithelium do, in the large majority of cases, reflect the overall tissue pattern and degree of cervical intraepithelial neoplasia.

NUCLEAR FEATURES

The nuclear changes in dyskaryosis are summarized in Table 2.5. Nuclear enlargement and chromatin aberration are always present, but not all features are invariably seen.

Nuclear enlargement

This is an essential feature of all dyskaryotic cells. However, not all cells where the nuclear area is much larger than the cytoplasmic area are dyskaryotic; differentiation must be made between dyskaryosis and those cells arising from an area of immature metaplasia (Fig. 2.20) or an atrophic, postmenopausal epithelium (Fig. 2.21).

A postpartum immature pattern can give rise to similar problems of interpretation. However, if due attention is paid to other more diagnostic features misinterpretation should not occur, although immature squamous metaplasia remains the most significant area of cytological misdiagnosis.

Irregular chromatin distribution

This is probably the most important single criterion used in the diagnosis of dyskaryosis (Fig. 2.22). An irregular distribution of chromatin with clumping throughout the nucleus is always present, and very often the nucleus has an irregular shape with indentations and, sometimes, protrusions (Fig. 2.23). Irregular thickening and prominence of the nuclear membrane can also be an important feature (see Fig. 2.23).

Hyperchromasia

Hyperchromasia (increased intensity of staining) is nearly always a prominent feature of dyskaryotic cells. However, it is not an essential feature, and dyskaryotic cells that are not more darkly stained than the normal cells associated with them may be overlooked by the inexperienced and unwary screener.

Mitotic figures

In cytological preparations, mitotic figures are rarely seen, even in CIN 3. This is a finding that lends support to the assumption that only cells from the top layers of epithelium are normally present in most cervical smears. Mitotic figures are, in fact, more frequently seen in association with regenerative changes. It is generally true that the more severe the degree of dyskaryosis, the more pronounced the nuclear features tend to be, although this correlation is not invariable.

Nucleoli

Nucleoli are not an important feature in the identification of dyskaryotic cells, and are virtually never present. Very occasionally small nucleoli may be seen, but these are not a prominent feature of dyskaryosis. Nucleoli are more usually found in regenerative changes.

Fig. 2.20 Immature squamous metaplasia. A tight group of cells with enlarged but fairly regular nuclei. Some hyperchromasia is present, but nuclear chromatin is bland and evenly distributed, with regular and even nuclear membranes. The cytoplasm appears thick and homogeneous, with a recognizable squamous shape.

Fig. 2.21 Severe dyskaryosis. A single, severely dyskaryotic cell, although showing hyperchromasia, is easily missed among large numbers of pale staining, normal parabasal cells in a postmenopausal atrophic pattern.

Fig. 2.22 Moderate dyskaryosis. A single binucleate cell, although the nuclei are pale stained and are not showing hyperchromasia; the chromatin is irregularly distributed, and the nuclei are irregular in shape.

Fig. 2.23 Mild to moderate dyskaryosis. Very large, pale nuclei but irregularly clumped chromatin, variation in size and shape, with irregularly thickened nuclear membranes.

CYTOPLASMIC CHANGES

By themselves, cytoplasmic changes are considerably less important in the identification of dyskaryotic cells than the nuclear changes described above. On the other hand, the amount of cytoplasm in relation to the size of nucleus is one of the most important considerations in assessing the degree of dyskaryosis. The lower the nuclear cytoplasmic ratio, the better differentiated the cell will be, and the milder the degree of dyskaryosis. This implies that individual cell differentiation is suggestive of a better organized and orientated epithelium. On the whole this is true, but there are exceptions.

The staining reaction which results in either acidophilic (pink staining) or basophilic (blue staining) cytoplasm may correspond to normal superficial and intermediate cell types, indicating mild or moderate dyskaryosis. However, this should not be regarded as a reliable criterion (Figs 2.24–2.27).

Keratinization

Keratinization of the cytoplasm can be seen in various situations, and cells showing keratinization must be carefully evaluated by close reference to nuclear features. In the context of cervical intraepithelial neoplasia, keratinization can be associated with all degrees of dyskaryosis (Fig 2.28), but it is also an important feature of human papillomavirus infection which may or may not coexist with all degrees of dyskaryosis. At the other end of the spectrum, atypical keratinization may be found in patients with invasive squamous cell carcinoma; attention to cellular shapes, as well as the arrangement of plaques and sheets of anucleate keratinized squamous cells, may assist in making a differential diagnosis.

Fig. 2.24 Moderate dyskaryosis. Typical basophilic stained cytoplasm, with enlarged hyperchromatic nuclei showing variation in nuclear size and shape.

Fig. 2.25 Mild dyskaryosis. Cells are showing typical nuclear features of dyskaryosis, with hyperchromasia and irregular chromatin clumping, enlarged and variously shaped nuclei. The cytoplasm is well defined and ample.

Fig. 2.26 Mild dyskaryosis. Prominent hyperchromatic nuclei, with ill defined cell borders. The spacing between the nuclei suggests a well preserved nuclear cytoplasmic ratio consistent with mild dyskaryosis.

Fig. 2.27 Mild dyskaryosis. Degeneration and karyorrhexis are seen on one cell. The thick, pink staining cytoplasm suggests maturation, consistent with mild dyskaryosis.

Fig. 2.28 Severe dyskaryosis with keratinization. (a) Loosely arranged sheet of cells, some with highly keratinized cytoplasm. **(b)** Large, severely dyskaryotic cells, with pale but grossly abnormal nuclei, closely associated with anucleate, keratinized, squamous cells.

Mixed degrees of dyskaryosis in a smear

Frequently, a cervical smear may contain a mixture of cells showing a variety of degrees of dyskaryosis (Figs 2.29 and 2.30), and a great deal of subjectivity is involved in assessing the overall dyskaryosis of a smear. This results in a discrepancy of opinion among cytologists, in the same way that differences of opinion exist among histopathologists.

A smear containing dyskaryotic cells of mainly moderate degree, with only one or two severely dyskaryotic cells, most probably reflects CIN 2. Conversely, if a smear contains the same small number of severely dyskaryotic cells, but none of any other degree of dyskaryosis, it almost certainly reflects CIN 3.

Fig. 2.29 Severe dyskaryosis. The typical, loosely associated sheets of cells are showing severe nuclear features with hyperchromasia, marked variations in size and shape of nuclei, with irregular chromatin pattern and variation in intensity of staining.

Fig. 2.30 Moderate and severe dyskaryosis. (a) Note the contrast between the cells at the top left of the field, which show moderate dyskaryosis with hyperchromatic nuclei and darkly stained cytoplasm, and the loose sheet of cells in the bottom right hand corner, which show severe dyskaryosis with large pale nuclei but the same degree of pleomorphism. **(b)** Many nuclei appear flattened and elongated, suggesting surface differentiation. Although the nuclei are not round as in most cases, the nuclear features are clearly those of dyskaryosis.

Dyskaryotic cells are often present in loosely associated streaks or small sheets of cells, as well as in large cohesive clumps (Figs 2.31–2.33); the latter appearance is more frequently seen in CIN 3. The quality of the smear in terms of thickness of cell spread, and the presence of physiological or degenerate changes, may also lead to difficulties in interpretation. On occasion, individual dyskaryotic cells may sometimes be seen, and once again it must be emphasized that careful and conscientious screening is of paramount importance if such cells are not to be completely overlooked (see Fig. 2.21; Fig. 2.34). Experience clearly plays an important role, and close liaison between cytologist, histopathologist and colposcopist can do much to improve expertise in all three disciplines.

With regard to patient management, differentiation between the various degrees of dyskaryosis and cervical intraepithelial neoplasia may not be important. However, in practical terms, it is a good discipline for cytologists to improve their ability to discriminate between various degrees of cellular change. This will enable them to make more critical assessments of the important areas of minimal invasion and glandular abnormalities, where subtle cellular changes are often the only indication of a more significant lesion which may require an alternative method of investigation and therapy.

Fig. 2.31 Severe dyskaryosis. The cells are characterized by marked pleomorphism and hyperchromasia.

Fig. 2.32 Severe dyskaryosis. Although the dyskaryotic cells can be evaluated and show the features of hyperchromasia and nuclear irregularity, the cytolytic nature of the smear (the result in this case of an exaggerated oral contraceptive effect) makes the background untidy and obscures cellular detail.

Fig. 2.33 Severe dyskaryosis. (a) Example of tight clusters of severely dyskaryotic cells which are sometimes seen. Piling up of the nuclei, results in some cells being out of focus. Variation in size and shape is best seen in the cells on the right. **(b)** The severely dyskaryotic cells in some instances show hyperchromasia, but others, particularly the two cells at the top of the string on the right, do not appear hyperchromatic. In addition, degenerative changes, such as pyknosis and karyorrhexis, confuse the pattern.

DIFFERENTIAL DIAGNOSIS OF CERVICAL INTRAEPITHELIAL NEOPLASIA

Although the histological diagnosis of cervical intraepithelial neoplasia is very often unequivocal, there are several conditions that can be confused with it, particularly the less severe degrees. Each of these epithelial states is described in detail in other chapters. Only those features relevant to their distinction from cervical intraepithelial neoplasia will be emphasized here.

Also, in cytological terms, discrimination between intraepithelial neoplasia and other cellular changes is obviously important, and a few areas consistently give rise to difficulty.

Immature squamous metaplasia

HISTOLOGY

By the very nature of its immaturity, this epithelial change has little or no surface differentiation or stratification, and because of this feature it may be confused with cervical intraepithelial neoplasia (Fig. 2.35). Furthermore, the cells of an active metaplasia frequently have an increased nuclear cytoplasmic ratio, with prominent nucleoli (see Fig. 2.35).

However, a distinction is usually possible by examining the nuclear detail: the nuclei of metaplastic cells are regular, both in shape and size, and may be hypochromatic rather than hyperchromatic. Mitotic figures may be present, but these are few in number and never show abnormal forms. Squamous metaplasia may involve crypts, but does so less often than cervical intraepithelial neoplasia.

CYTOLOGY

When cells from a maturing area of squamous metaplasia are seen in the smear, few problems are likely to arise, but cells arising from an area of very immature squamous metaplasia may give rise to misinterpretation. The nuclei are always enlarged and frequently have an active and hyperchromatic pattern. However, the chromatin distribution is regular, with a finely granular background matrix. The nuclear membrane is even and finely circumscribed, with no thickening or indentation (see Fig. 2.20).

Congenital transformation zone

HISTOLOGY

This is a variant of squamous metaplasia; the epithelium of the congenital transformation zone is composed of maturing metaplastic cells (see pages 78 and 79 for the colposcopic appearances). There is often a little hyperkeratosis on the surface, but the most alarming feature for the unwary pathologist is the irregular pattern of the basement membrane (Fig. 2.36). This gives the appearance of random, spiky downgrowths of squamous cells into the stroma; to increase the confusion, the centres of these processes may contain whorls of more mature cells. As with squamous metaplasia, the regularity of nuclei and lack of mitotic activity help to distinguish the congenital transformation zone from cervical intraepithelial neoplasia.

Having established that the epithelium does not show the features of intraepithelial neoplasia, irregularity of the epithelial/stromal junction ceases to be alarming.

Fig. 2.34 A single severely dyskaryotic cell. This is discretely placed among normal mature squamous cells (arrow).

Fig. 2.35 Immature squamous metaplasia. There is significant arrest of maturation, with large nuclei of the basal half of the epithelium. Despite this increased nuclear/cytoplasmic ratio, the nuclei are regular and mitotic figures are very infrequent. H & E, × 128.

Fig. 2.36 Congenital transformation zone. Keratinization is present on the surface, and the characteristic irregular pattern of the epithelial stromal junction is seen. H&E, × 32.

CYTOLOGY

Cells arising from a congenital transformation zone have no cytological features to distinguish them from any other area of metaplasia.

Healing epithelium

HISTOLOGY

After local destructive treatment for cervical intraepithelial neoplasia, it is common to encounter areas of acetowhite epithelium at colposcopic follow up. The colposcopist may feel that the appearances are those of residual disease, and will therefore take a biopsy (see Chapter 7).

The histological features of this epithelium are very similar to those of squamous metaplasia, with lack of maturation and large, pale nuclei (Fig. 2.37). It is important that these changes are recognized and not mistaken for cervical intraepithelial neoplasia, although it is equally important not to miss the latter and underdiagnose it as healing epithelium.

In healing epithelium, it is also quite common to find evidence of human papillomavirus infection. With a little experience, distinguishing between this type of epithelium and minor degrees of residual cervical intraepithelial neoplasia becomes easier, if attention is paid to the lack of nuclear abnormalities and sparseness of mitotic figures.

CYTOLOGY

Cells arising from areas of regeneration or repair are likely to show active and hyperchromatic nuclei, but careful evaluation of chromatin distribution, shape and size of nuclei will, in most instances, successfully resolve any difficulties (Fig. 2.38).

Subclinical papillomavirus infection

HISTOLOGY

One of the hallmarks of subclinical papillomavirus infection is koilocytotic change in the cell: the nucleus becomes irregular, hyperchromatic and enlarged,

Fig. 2.37 Healing after laser vaporization. The appearances are very similar to those of immature squamous metaplasia. Occasional mitotic figures may be seen, and there is nuclear enlargement. H&E, × 32.

Fig. 2.38 Regeneration and repair. Large, hyperchromatic nuclei are granular, but chromatin is regularly distributed throughout the nuclei; nuclear membranes are even and regular.

surrounded by an exaggerated perinuclear halo. At low magnification, epithelium containing many cells showing koilocytotic change gives the impression of widespread nuclear enlargement and irregularity, which may lead to an erroneous diagnosis of cervical intraepithelial neoplasia. In assessing whether or not an epithelium showing subclinical papillomavirus infection also contains cervical intraepithelial neoplasia, the cells not showing koilocytotic change must be evaluated. If these show no more than a minimal variation in size and shape, a diagnosis of cervical intraepithelial neoplasia is not justified.

Furthermore, subclinical papillomavirus infection can cause an increase in the number of mitotic figures in the epithelium, therefore the presence of mitotic figures cannot be taken as evidence of cervical intraepithelial neoplasia if the other features of subclinical papillomavirus are also seen.

Very frequently, cervical intraepithelial neoplasia and subclinical papillomavirus infection coexist in the same area of epithelium; in this case, the presence of the latter must not be taken as an explanation for the nuclear changes which may be present as a manifestation of a genuine cervical intraepithelial neoplasia.

CYTOLOGY

The cellular features associated with human papillomavirus infection are discussed in detail in Chapter 12. Here, it is important to stress that whenever the nuclear features of dyskaryosis are present, the cell must be regarded as such and reported accordingly, whether or not the other features of human papillo-

mavirus infection are seen in that particular cell or in associated cells (Fig. 2.39).

Atrophic postmenopausal epithelium

HISTOLOGY

If the oestrogenic stimulus, which encourages the squamous epithelium of the cervix to mature, is withdrawn, the epithelium becomes thin and atrophic. It is only a few cells thick, and the nuclear cytoplasmic ratio increases. However, this process is the opposite of that occurring in cervical intraepithelial neoplasia: it is the cytoplasm that is reduced in amount, rather than the nucleus that is increased.

The results of these changes may give an appearance that can be very difficult to distinguish from cervical intraepithelial neoplasia, with large nuclei occupying a significant proportion of the epithelium (Fig. 2.40).

Mitotic figures are not seen in an atrophic epithelium, and an experienced pathologist will recognize that the nuclei are smaller than those found in cervical intraepithelial neoplasia. Nevertheless, an atrophic epithelium can often give rise to difficulties in interpretation, particularly when it is found on a small cervical or vault biopsy.

Fig. 2.39 Moderate and severe dyskaryosis with human papillomavirus changes. Quite marked pleomorphism of the nuclei is seen. Also seen are dyskeratosis, with keratinization and occasional koilocytotic change, characteristic of papillomavirus infection.

Fig. 2.40 Atrophic postmenopausal epithelium. The nuclei appear large, but this is due to loss of cytoplasm and not an increase in nuclear size. Hyperchromasia is present, but no mitotic activity is seen. H&E, × 128.

CYTOLOGY

Cells arising from an atrophic epithelium are easily recognized, as the nuclei are often very pale, with a fine chromatin pattern (Fig. 2.41). However, in the presence of infection the nuclei may appear more active, and such smears remain a source of error leading to a false positive diagnosis.

Equally important is a false negative diagnosis which may result when dyskaryotic cells are mistaken for normal parabasal cells. Postpartum patterns may also give rise to the same problems of differential diagnosis.

Endometrial cells

CYTOLOGY

Endometrial cells may occasionally be mistaken for severely dyskaryotic cells in a smear, particularly when degenerative changes give rise to darkly stained nuclei, or where nuclear changes associated with an intrauterine contraceptive device are seen (Fig. 2.42). In the latter case, the enlarged and active-looking nuclei can be difficult to interpret, but careful attention to other nuclear features and the cytoplasm, as well as the overall smear pattern, will usually resolve the issue.

On rare occasions, it may be impossible to distinguish between cells arising from an area of CIN 3 and endocervical (or endometrial) carcinoma.

Fig. 2.41 Atrophic postmenopausal pattern. Parabasal cells showing degenerative changes, particularly swelling, bloating and nuclear distortion. Numerous polymorphs, together with pyknosis and karyorrhexis, are frequently seen.

Fig. 2.42 Endometrial cells associated with the use of an intrauterine contraceptive device. Occasional discrete cells show darkly staining nuclei. Although chromatin is clumped, the background matrix is finely granular. These cells are typical endometrial cells of glandular type. Large cells, at the lower centre, are probably stromal and show reactive changes.

ADDENDUM

Proposed modifications to cytological and histological terminology

CYTOLOGICAL CLASSIFICATION

In 1989, the National Cancer Institute published a statement recommending a new approach to the reporting of cervical and vaginal smears, which has become known as the 'Bethesda Classification'. Its development resulted from a perceived need to reclassify the terminology in order to relate it, in a more meaningful way than previously, to patient management.

In addition, it was hoped that a new approach to terminology might improve communication between cytopathologists, as well as between cytopathologists and clinicians.

The Bethesda classification discards the Papanicolaou grading system (as does the British Society for Clinical Cytology classification presented above), because it is not related to modern diagnostic cytological practice. It also rejects an association with the CIN terminology, due to its lack of reproducibility between different pathologists, and because it does not offer clear management guidelines.

The Bethesda classification attempts to overcome the shortcomings of other systems of classification, by using a detailed system that may be abbreviated as follows:
1. Within normal limits.
2. Atypia, not classifiable elsewhere.
3. Cellular changes suggesting:
   (a) A low grade squamous intraepithelial lesion;
   (b) A high grade squamous intraepithelial lesion.

Additional comments can be made regarding the presence of human papillomavirus changes (these are put into the low grade category, even when no features of intraepithelial neoplasia are seen) and the presence or absence of glandular cells, squamous metaplastic cell components.

The main advantage of this classification is that it links the cytological report to a management policy, in that lesions reported as being of high grade require colposcopy and treatment, whereas those of low grade may be managed more conservatively.

However, the proposal of this new terminology does give the impression of change for its own sake as, whatever system of classification is employed, there will be a need for borderlines to be defined; in this case, between low and high grade lesions: no help is given as to how this breakpoint is identified.

Further criticisms are that the reintroduction of the term 'atypical' seems to be a retrograde step because of its imprecision, and also that the terminology employs what are essentially histological terms; the BSCC believes that cytologists should use cytological terms.

The Bethesda classification has no advantages over the BSCC terminology which has been presented in detail earlier in this Chapter. The latter terminology links the cytology report to the management policy for the patient and is more meaningful in practical terms, as well as more flexible in allowing adjustments that may be required to fit in with local considerations.

Furthermore, it fully addresses the dilemmas of persistent minor changes and the unsatisfactory smear. It disregards the inadequate term 'atypical', it uses cytological rather than histological terms, and can be readily adapted to relate to low and high risk cellular changes, if the point in the spectrum of dyskaryosis at which cellular changes progress from low to high risk can be determined.

HISTOLOGICAL CLASSIFICATION

New approaches to the histological classification of intraepithelial neoplasia, closely paralleling the Bethesda cytological classification, have been proposed, on the basis that its subdivision into three categories is artificial. It has been proposed that cervical intraepithelial neoplasia should be split into two categories only: low grade and high grade lesions.

Richart suggests that the conceptual breakpoint should come between those minor lesions that have no evidence of aneuploidy and are associated with a heterogeneous group of human papillomavirus types, and those that have abnormal mitotic figures, indicating aneuploidy, and contain high and intermediate risk human papillomavirus types.

The latter group of lesions (CIN 2 and CIN 3) are considered to be precursors of invasive carcinoma, whereas the former (CIN 1 with human papillomavirus related changes) have an unpredictable outcome.

This view is a restatement of the long accepted, pragmatic approach to the subdivision of cervical intraepithelial neoplasia into those lesions which have a high risk of progression to invasion, and those which apparently have a low risk. This can be linked to a sensible approach to treatment.

However, as with cytology, there remains a dividing line between the low grade and high grade lesions; therefore, no matter how attractive this concept may seem in theory, practical difficulties will persist in determining the borderline and in allocating lesions which fall near the borderline.

Moreover, the value of an approach that relies, even partly, on the presence and type of human papillomavirus infection is questionable.

REFERENCES

Richart, R. M. (1990 A Modified Terminolgy for Cervical Intraepithelial Neoplasia. *Obstetrics and Gynecology,* **75**, 131–3.

Robertson, A. J., Anderson, J. M., Swanson-Beck, J. *et al.* (1989) Observer Variability in Histopathological Reporting of Cervical Biopsy Specimens. *Journal of Clinical Pathology,* **42,** 231–8.

The 1988 Bethesda System for Reporting Cervical/ Vaginal Cytological Diagnoses (1985) *Journal of the American Medical Association,* **262,** 931–4.

3. Aetiology and Natural History of Cervical Carcinoma

INTRODUCTION

Squamous cell carcinoma of the cervix and its precursors have been widely investigated, and much has been written about their epidemiology and aetiology. A number of epidemiological factors that appear to contribute to the development of a neoplasm have been identified, but the way in which these factors relate to the causative agent, or agents, is not yet clear.

More importantly, these aetiological agents have not been identified conclusively, although different types of agents have been incriminated from time to time.

Changes in the cervix and interreactions of aetiological agents in the development of cervical carcinoma are summarized in Fig. 3.1.

EPIDEMIOLOGY

The results of a large number of epidemiological studies comparing women with the disease with those who do not have the disease, are summarized below. Some studies have looked at invasive cancer as 'the disease', others have considered cervical intraepithelial neoplasia, whilst a number of them have looked at both invasive cancer and cervical intraepithelial neoplasia.

The results appear to be broadly similar in all three groups. Naturally, these studies do not agree in all respects, but the findings discussed here represent the results of the majority in each case.

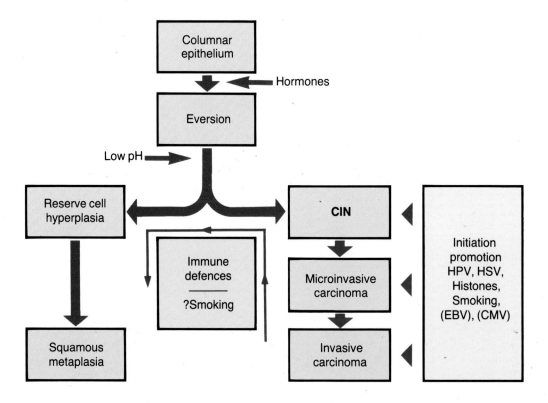

Fig. 3.1 Actions and interactions in the development of cervical carcinoma. Hormonally induced eversion of the cervix and an acidic vaginal environment encourage the development of the transformation zone (see pages 14 and 15). In physiological conditions, benign squamous metaplasia is the eventual outcome. In the presence of a sexually transmitted agent, the benign metaplastic process is diverted into a malignant transformation, resulting first in increasingly severe grades of cervical intraepithelial neoplasia and then, in an unknown proportion of women, invasive squamous cell carcinoma. A number of carcinogens are suggested here. Whether the agents act in unison or sequentially as initiators and promoters is also

unclear, and it is not known whether continued exposure to the carcinogen (or another agent) is necessary for the progression of cervical intraepithelial neoplasia from mild to severe degrees, or for the establishment of an invasive carcinoma. It is unlikely that local and systemic immune defences are important in counteracting the changes generated by the carcinogenic agents, at the stage of development of cervical intraepithelial neoplasia, during its progression through the different grades, at the point of beginning invasion and at the time when a microinvasive carcinoma expands to become established as stage Ib carcinoma with metastatic potential.

Coitus

Squamous cell carcinoma of the cervix does not occur in women who have never had sexual intercourse; coitus is the major prerequisite for the development of this tumour.

In the past, extensive investigations of medical records and death certificates of nuns showed how rare cervical cancer of any type was in a group of women who were assumed never to have had sexual intercourse.

Age at first coitus

Several epidemiological studies have shown that women with cervical cancer are more likely to have become sexually active during adolescence, than matched controls without the disease.

Age at marriage and age at first pregnancy have also been looked at, and similar results have been observed. These factors obviously reflect the age at first intercourse.

Number of partners

Many investigations have indicated that women with cervical cancer and precancer are more likely to have had extramarital partners than control groups without the disease. In fact, promiscuity in either sex increases the risk of cervical cancer.

Frequency of coitus

There is no evidence that frequency of intercourse is a significant factor, provided that this does not imply a greater number of partners.

Parity

It has been apparent for many years that women with cervical cancer tend to have more children than women without the disease. However, when the obvious correlation between high parity and an early age at marriage is taken into consideration, this association between high parity and carcinoma of the cervix disappears.

It seems that high parity reflects sexual activity starting at an early age; the suggestion that the birth of several children repeatedly traumatizes the cervix, with trauma predisposing to the development of malignancy, is unfounded.

Sexually transmitted diseases

Women with cervical cancer have a high frequency of sexually transmitted diseases (syphilis, gonorrhoea, trichomoniasis, genital herpes, papillomavirus infection and *Chlamydia* infection).

It is possible that all these infections are related to the tumour, but only in the sense that they are a consequence of intercourse, as is cervical cancer, and therefore have a common epidemiological background. However, some of these infections have been incriminated as causative agents, and will be discussed in more detail below.

Male circumcision

There has been a long standing belief that circumcision of the male protects the female from developing cervical cancer. This belief was established partly because of the low incidence of cervical cancer in Jewish women, and partly as the result of two totally uncontrolled epidemiological studies carried out in the 1940s.

One of these studies demonstrated a lower incidence of cervical cancer among native Fijian women, compared with immigrant Hindu women in the same country.

The second study compared the incidence of cervical cancer in Hindu and Muslim women in India, finding a higher incidence in the Hindu than in the Muslim population. It was suggested that the differences found in both these investigations were the result of circumcision of Fijian and Muslim men.

A number of subsequent studies have repeated these investigations, using controls for as many other factors as possible, but they give no support to the suggestion that male circumcision protects from cervical cancer.

Racial factors

The interrelationship between racial, cultural and religious factors in the development of cervical cancer is illustrated by reference to cervical cancer in Jewish women, who have repeatedly been shown to have a low incidence of the disease.

However, this apparent partial immunity may be related more to the regulation of sexual life by observing the laws of Niddah, than to circumcision of the male or a hereditary resistance to the disease. Therefore, low incidence is probably due to the fact that orthodox Jews tend not to have intercourse during adolescence, and not to have multiple sexual partners. There is some evidence to suggest that the incidence of cervical cancer is higher in Jewish women who adhere less rigidly to this strict sexual code.

Socioeconomic factors

Epidemiological studies in the past have shown that women from lower socioeconomic groups have a higher incidence of cervical cancer, than those in the higher income groups. The reason for this is obscure but, again, it is possible that an early age at first intercourse and marriage may be the most important factor.

However, no association has been demonstrated between social class and the risk of developing cervical intraepithelial neoplasia.

Smoking

It has recently become apparent that there is an important correlation between cigarette smoking and the risk of developing cervical intraepithelial neoplasia and cervical carcinoma. This finding was initially explained away by the supposition that young women who smoked were more likely to have intercourse at an early age, and to have multiple partners. Subsequent, carefully controlled, epidemiological studies have indicated that this was a false assumption, and that the risk from cigarette smoking is maintained after controlling for all other factors.

It remains to be shown whether cigarette smoking acts by a local carcinogenic or co-carcinogenic effect, or by suppression of local immune mechanisms in the cervix.

Method of contraception

There have been several major epidemiological studies investigating whether or not there is an association between oral contraceptive use and increased risk of cervical neoplasia, with conflicting results.

The main difficulty with these studies is that a woman's choice of contraceptive method may depend on other factors which influence the possibility of developing cervical cancer. For instance, women who use different methods of contraception are likely to have different attitudes to sexual behaviour.

A small number of well controlled epidemiological studies have indicated that the risk of developing cervical cancer increases in proportion to the length of oral contraceptive use. Rather than incriminating a direct effect of the contraceptive pill, it could be argued that the rate of cervical precancer has been increasing in parallel with the growing popularity of this form of contraception, and that this increase can be explained by a change in sexual behaviour.

Furthermore, progestagens cause eversion of the cervix, which enables endocervical lesions to be more readily diagnosed.

Another factor which may bias the results of studies is that women taking oral contraceptives possibly have more frequent cervical smears.

The use of barrier methods of contraception should protect the cervical epithelium from an agent transmitted at intercourse, if it is assumed that cervical cancer is caused by an infective agent. A number of studies have shown that women who consistently use barrier methods of contraception have approximately one-quarter of the risk of cervical neoplasia, compared with women who use other methods of contraception.

Male factors

The only satisfactory explanation of the importance of intercourse in the development of cervical cancer is that an agent of some description is transmitted from the male to the female at intercourse. If this agent is carried by some men but not by others, then the woman who is promiscuous is more likely to encounter a man who is a carrier.

If the agent is carried by both sexes and can be transmitted from a female carrier (not necessarily a woman who is developing cervical cancer) to a male, then the chances of a man being a carrier are proportional to the number of his partners. This would mean that a woman who has intercourse with a promiscuous man, although he may be her only sexual partner, is at risk of developing cervical cancer by his promiscuity.

Support for this hypothesis is provided by studies showing that the incidence of the tumour may be related to the occupation of the patient's partner, in a way which does not necessarily reflect socioeconomic status but which may be linked with opportunities for promiscuity in the man.

Immunological factors

Cervical intraepithelial neoplasia and invasive cancer are more common in women who are immunosuppressed; a 14-fold increase in the incidence of CIN 3 has been demonstrated in renal transplant recipients. This increased risk may be the result of impaired immunological surveillance, so that malignant cellular changes are not recognized and tumours can develop unchecked.

Alternatively, it is possible that resistance to mutagenic viruses is lowered; this point may be particularly relevant to the cervix, in view of the possible role of viruses in the aetiology of cervical cancer.

A third possibility is that immunosuppressive drugs are carcinogenic. Studies on local immune mechanisms within the cervix reveal that an inadequate host response may play a part in allowing progression to cervical intraepithelial neoplasia, after the external mutagen has been encountered.

TRANSMISSIBLE AGENTS

From the above discussions it appears that the development of cervical cancer and its precursors almost certainly depends on the transmission of an agent, or agents, from one individual to another. Therefore, it is now relevant to consider what these agents may be.

Over the years, a large number of substances which could be transmitted from a man to a woman at intercourse have been considered. All of these have, at different times, been put forward as possible causes of cervical cancer. Only a few of them will be discussed here.

Smegma

The question whether male circumcision protects the woman from cervical cancer has been considered above. The possibility that this factor was linked with a reduced risk of the disease in the female partners of circumcised men, rested largely with the assumption that smegma may be a chemical carcinogen.

Smegma has also been incriminated as a factor responsible for the higher incidence of this tumour in the lower socioeconomic groups, and in this respect it has been linked to poor cleanliness. However, there is no evidence that human smegma is carcinogenic.

Nevertheless, there seems to be a genuine relationship between absence of circumcision and increased risk of developing penile carcinoma. Furthermore, there is evidence that the wives of men with penile cancer are at greater risk of developing cervical cancer, which suggests a remote but real association.

Spermatozoa

Spermatozoa are packed with deoxyribonucleic acid (DNA), very closely related to the DNA of the metaplastic endocervical cell. Because of this, spermatozoa could be considered a prime suspect for causing mutagenic DNA interactions. Some evidence has shown that endocervical cells are capable of phagocytosing sperm heads, but integration of sperm and endocervical cell DNA has not been demonstrated.

Basic proteins

The possible role of spermatozoa in the aetiology of cervical cancer was further investigated by examining the protein content in sperm rather than its DNA content, and superficial contact with the endocervical cell rather than entry into it.

It was suggested that an arginine-rich histone in the sperm head had an effect on DNA filaments originating from the nuclear DNA, which, while remaining connected with the nucleus, protruded through the cell surface. These filaments in the mucoid coat may act as a 'switch-gear' which, if suitably stimulated, activates the DNA within the cell, resulting in an increased capacity for protein synthesis and proliferation (both of which are characteristics of cancer cells).

Chlamydia

Chlamydia trachomatis is a common pathogen, causing chronic infection of the cervix and fallopian tubes. As with many other sexually transmitted infective agents, it is reasonable to consider that *Chlamydia* may perhaps play a part in cervical carcinogenesis.

There is an association between infection with *Chlamydia* and cervical precancer: a higher prevalence of positive cultures and serum antibodies to *Chlamydia* has been shown in women with cervical intraepithelial neoplasia, together with a higher incidence of *Chlamydia*-associated changes in smears, compared with controls. In addition, a higher progression rate to CIN 3 has been seen in women with chlamydial changes in their smears than in a control group of women without such changes.

However, these findings may only be due to the fact that both diseases are the consequence of sexual intercourse.

Viruses

HERPES SIMPLEX VIRUS TYPE 2 (HSV–2)

Women with cervical cancer have an increased incidence of HSV-2 antibodies, compared with women who have non-malignant gynaecological complaints. Furthermore, HSV-2 is capable of transforming cells in tissue culture.

However, HSV-2 DNA has only rarely been found in tumour samples (Fig. 3.2). Further evidence against HSV-2 being related to cervical neoplasia has come from studies demonstrating that the incidence of HSV-2 antibodies is more closely related to sexual behaviour than to the presence of neoplasia.

41

HUMAN PAPILLOMAVIRUS

Since the mid-1970s, human papillomavirus infection (Fig. 3.3) has been at the centre of investigations into the aetiology of cervical cancer. Many studies have shown that a high proportion of cervical tumours contain HPV-DNA, in particular HPV-16, HPV-18 and HPV-33.

Furthermore, cervical intraepithelial neoplasia is very frequently found in association with morphological features indicative of human papillomavirus infection (see Chapter 12). Studies involving immunocytochemistry (Fig. 3.4) and DNA–DNA hybridization on such specimens have confirmed with sufficient certainty that these appearances, recognized under the light microscope after routine processing and staining, are indeed the result of infection by human papillomavirus.

The inability to culture the virus in the laboratory has led to a system of viral typing based on DNA homology rather than serology, and over 60 different human papillomavirus types have now been reported. Once the cell is infected, the virus persists in the nucleus as circular DNA, referred to as 'episomal', which is distinct from the cellular DNA.

Analysis of the genomes has shown that the viral DNA may be divided into regions, the early and late regions being of most interest. The segment of DNA between the end of late proteins and the start of early proteins contains a number of DNA sequences which are thought to be of importance in controlling viral protein synthesis and replication. In addition, it has been found that the regions encoding the E6 and E7 proteins of HPV-16 and HPV-18 are capable of immortalizing and transforming tissue cells in culture, and it seems that in HPV-16 the E7 protein has the maximum ability to transform cells.

Human papillomavirus infection of the cervix may be subdivided into two groups: HPV-6, HPV-11, HPV-31 and HPV-35 are thought to be associated with condylomata acuminata, low grade intraepithelial neoplasia, and only rarely with invasive tumours.

HPV-16, HPV-18 and HPV-33 are associated with subclinical papillomavirus infection, low grade cervical intraepithelial neoplasia which progresses, high grade intraepithelial neoplasia and invasive carcinomas. It is this latter group of human papillomavirus types that has the ability to transform cells in culture, and to cooperate with oncogenes in cellular transformation.

It has been shown that the majority of cervical tumours contain a proportion of HPV-DNA which,

Fig. 3.2 Invasive squamous carcinoma of the cervix. Immunofluorescence using a monoclonal antibody to a herpes simplex virus-specific protein. Cancer cells are positive.

Fig. 3.3 TEM koilocyte from a cervical human papillomavirus-induced lesion. Crystalline or 'honeycomb' patterns of human papillomavirus particles are seen (left and right).

Fig. 3.4 Cervical intraepithelial neoplasia. Immunoperoxidase method for human papillomavirus-associated protein. A positive reaction (brown staining) in the koilocytes is seen near the surface of abnormal epithelium.

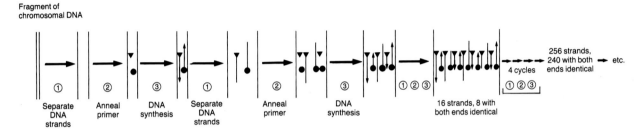

Fig. 3.5 The polymerase chain reaction for amplifying specific nucleotide sequences in vitro. (a) DNA isolated from cells is heated to separate its complementary strands. These strands are then annealed with an excess of two DNA oligonucleotides (each 15–20 nucleotides long) which have been chemically synthesized to match sequences separated by x nucleotides (where x is generally between 50 and 2000). The two oligonucleotides serve as specific primers for in vitro DNA synthesis catalysed by DNA polymerase, which copies the DNA between the sequences corresponding to the two oligonucleotides. **(b)** After multiple cycles of reaction, a large amount of a single DNA fragment, x nucleotides long, is obtained, provided that the original DNA sample contains the DNA sequence that was anticipated when the two oligonucleotides were designed.

instead of being episomal, is integrated within the host genome.

Prevalence and significance of human papillomavirus infection

The development of the polymerase chain reaction has resulted in great advances in the identification of human papillomavirus infection (Fig. 3.5). Hitherto, the detection of HPV-DNA was dependent on a minimum amount of DNA being available, and very small quantities could not be detected. The polymerase chain reaction amplifies DNA dramatically, so that very small quantities of DNA may now be identified.

Early investigations using this method have shown that HPV-DNA is, in fact, present in normal cervical tissue in many women. This high prevalence of human papillomavirus infection may suggest that the virus is merely an innocent passenger; it may also support the hypothesis that this infection is only one step in the process leading to cervical neoplasia.

It is very likely that cervical cancer is caused by a number of factors or agents, and has a multistep aetiology which requires initiation by one agent and promotion by another. It is probable that herpes simplex virus, human papillomavirus, smoking, and even other factors not yet considered, all act together or in succession, resulting in the evolution of the disease. Also, different aetiologies may be involved in different women.

NATURAL HISTORY OF CERVICAL CARCINOMA

In order to treat cervical intraepithelial neoplasia most effectively, it is necessary to have an understanding of the relationships between the various grades of cervical intraepithelial neoplasia, and also between cervical intraepithelial neoplasia and invasive carcinoma. A great deal of work has been done in an attempt to establish these relationships, but an accurate knowledge of the natural history of this disease still eludes us.

Progression of cervical intraepithelial neoplasia

There have been several studies of the apparent

progression from minor degrees of intraepithelial neoplasia to more severe degrees. Some of these studies have involved examination by colposcopy and cytology, whereas others have added the histology of biopsies.

In general, it has been shown that a mild or moderate degree of cervical intraepithelial neoplasia will either progress to a more severe form, or it will regress. Regression is more likely in the milder forms, and there is evidence that taking biopsies encourages this process, a fact that may invalidate prospective studies in which biopsies are taken at the beginning of or during the study.

It may be reasonable to assume that progression through the grades of cervical intraepithelial neoplasia occurs in a gradual, incremental fashion, but there is no direct evidence for this. Most of the studies that have shown a gradual progression have been sampling the cervix as a whole, either by cytology or by directed biopsies from the most abnormal areas. It is not possible to study a single small area of epithelium by biopsy over a period of time, as the biopsy removes the tissue being studied.

If, as is quite likely, cervical intraepithelial neoplasia represents abnormal clones of cells, a clone with abnormalities of severe degree may develop suddenly within a field of minor abnormality. Furthermore, the same argument can be used to suggest that severely abnormal degrees of intraepithelial neoplasia may develop without necessarily being preceded by minor abnormalities.

Relationship of cervical intraepithelial neoplasia to invasive carcinoma

The success of effective cervical screening programmes which detect cervical intraepithelial neoplasia by cytology and allow its treatment whilst still in the preinvasive phase, rests largely on two assumptions:

1. A significant proportion of women with cervical intraepithelial neoplasia would eventually develop invasive carcinoma, if not treated.
2. Most invasive squamous cell carcinomas are preceded by a demonstrable intraepithelial phase.

However, there is little precise information on the rate of progression from cervical intraepithelial neoplasia to invasive carcinoma, mainly because of the moral and ethical impossibility of observing women with a known premalignant disease without intervention. Even so, some figures are available from a number of studies.

In the 1950s, two studies from Scandinavia established progression rates of 65–70% in women with carcinoma in situ (CIN 3) who developed invasive

carcinoma over the course of up to 12 years. A more recent study from New Zealand found that 36% of women who had persistent abnormal cytology following incomplete treatment for CIN 3, developed invasive carcinoma after 20 years; 18% had developed carcinoma after 10 years.

This figure of 36% of women progressing to invasive carcinoma after 20 years is surprisingly low, but it must be remembered that those patients were partially treated, so that the disease was probably not allowed to run its natural course.

This illustrates the other main flaw of this type of study, namely, the inability to make a reliable diagnosis without removing tissue, which would interfere with the natural progression of the disease. Taken in correlation with the moral barrier to such a study, it seems very unlikely that precise figures for the rate of progression from cervical intraepithelial neoplasia to invasive carcinoma will ever be known.

Duration of the preinvasive phase

It has long been accepted from epidemiological and cytological studies that cervical intraepithelial neoplasia takes at least 10 years to become invasive, although more recent analyses indicate that 3–10 years may be more realistic. The fact that women with CIN 3 are generally some 10–15 years younger than those with invasive carcinoma, is taken to support this suggestion.

Nevertheless, there have been worrying reports of young women developing invasive carcinoma of the cervix following recent negative cytology. Some of these smears may have been genuine false negatives, which would have been found to contain malignant cells on review. However, it is impossible to escape the conclusion that, at least in some of these women, there had been a genuine progression from a normal cervix to invasive carcinoma during the short time, reported to be as little as six months, between the initial smear and subsequent diagnosis of carcinoma.

It may be reasonable to suggest that, although the mean time interval for progression through cervical intraepithelial neoplasia to invasive carcinoma may be 10–15 years, a small number of women will fall at the two extremes of the distribution curve of the length of natural history (Fig. 3.6). As a result, some women will have such a long natural history that progression to invasive disease will never occur in the course of a lifetime; these women would be classified as 'non-progressors'.

Equally, at the other end of the spectrum there will be some women in whom the natural history of the disease runs a very rapid course, measured in months rather than years; this may be the case

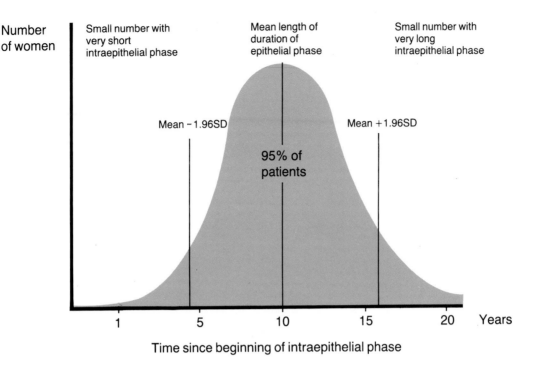

Number of women

Small number with very short intraepithelial phase

Mean length of duration of epithelial phase

Small number with very long intraepithelial phase

Mean – 1.96SD

Mean +1.96SD

95% of patients

Time since beginning of intraepithelial phase

Years

Fig. 3.6 Natural history of cervical intraepithelial neoplasia. The Gaussian curve represents the length of time during which the disease remains intraepithelial before it becomes invasive. It is assumed that duration of the intraepithelial phases in a population of women with cervical intraepithelial neoplasia follows a natural distribution. The mean has been arbitrarily taken to be 10 years; 95% of women will have a length of intraepithelial phase that falls within 1.96 standard deviations on either side of the mean.

At the two extreme ends of the curve, there will be women whose intraepithelial phase will be either very long (greater than a lifetime) or very short (weeks or months, rather than years). The curve has been intentionally skewed to lengthen it on the right, to allow for the apparently large number of women who either would not develop invasive disease at all, or would progress to invasive carcinoma only after several years.

described in the above reports.

This speculative suggestion reconciles the very diverse progression rates in different women, with the belief that one disease process is occurring. These differences in behaviour represent extreme variations in the length of the natural history of the same disease, and it is not necessary to suggest that rapidly progressing cervical cancer is a different disease.

CYTOLOGICAL INDICATIONS

The decision to refer a woman for colposcopic examination is based on a number of factors, of which by far the most important is the result of the cervical smear. However, consideration must also be given to the facilities available, and to the psychological impact of referral on the women concerned.

These factors play a part both in developing a policy for referral of women to a colposcopy clinic at a local or, preferably, national level, and in determining whether an individual woman should be referred

for the examination. Referral of women with very minor abnormalities could overload a clinic with limited resources, and thus jeopardize the prompt treatment of more severe abnormalities, if care is not taken to prioritize referrals.

For many women with minor abnormalities in their smears, the psychological effect of referral for colposcopy, with or without subsequent treatment, may be greater than the risk of serious disease developing from the abnormality that the smear has identified. It is an important requirement of a screening programme that overall it should do more good than harm to the population.

The smear result itself cannot be taken entirely at face value. Although most cytology departments quite rightly claim a good correlation between cytological findings and final histological diagnosis, it cannot always be assumed that a smear report of mild dyskaryosis means that only CIN 1 is present in the cervix. Several studies have shown that, within a group of women with smears reported as showing mild dyskaryosis, there is a proportion, perhaps as many as one-fifth to a quarter, who are found to have CIN 3 at colposcopy and biopsy.

On the other hand, an even larger proportion of women with mildly dyskaryotic smears have no demonstrable abnormality at colposcopy. Therefore, when deciding whether to refer a woman for colposcopy, it is necessary to bear in mind the possibility of more severe disease being present than the smear suggests, and to assess the probable natural history of the lesion that is predicted by cytology.

Whilst it is accepted that the need to repeat a cervical smear can cause anxiety to women, it has become clear that more anxiety may be caused by the referral for colposcopy and actual colposcopic examination.

The interests of the women concerned are best served by a balanced approach which takes into account not only the most satisfactory clinical management, but also the most effective use of resources in terms of cost and manpower.

It is important that the referral protocol is flexible enough to allow for temporary constraints of whatever nature, and also to tailor management to the needs of individual patients. Furthermore, adjustments need to be made with the changing pattern of understanding and knowledge of cervical intraepithelial neoplasia.

4. Indications for Referral for Colposcopy

APPROACH TO REFERRAL

The following model is based on a 'common sense' approach (Table 4.1). All women with cervical smears suggesting moderate or severe dyskaryosis, and those showing any suggestion of invasive disease or adenocarcinoma, should be referred immediately for colposcopy.

In the case of borderline changes, the current approach is to take another smear after six months. If at that time the changes persist, referral for colposcopy should be considered (see page 143).

There is a case for managing mild, and perhaps even moderate, dyskaryosis in the same way as borderline changes, especially if the cytological features of human papillomavirus infection are seen; these can confuse the picture, and lead to either underdiagnosis or overdiagnosis. Repeat smears at intervals may clarify the pattern, and if the abnormality persists on a second or, at most, a third smear, referral is advised.

The case of persistent unsatisfactory smears requires some special discussion (see Table 5.2). Unless some attempt is made to identify and treat the causative agents, there is little point in repeating smears ad infinitum. If the cytologist can give an indication that a bacterial infection is present, then microbiological screening would be indicated, with appropriate treatment. Should the smear remain unsatisfactory when repeated on no more than three occasions over a period (of, say, six to 12 months), then referral for colposcopy is justified.

Women taking the oral contraceptive pill form a special group, since some consistently present with a markedly cytolytic smear showing clumping and folding of cells, making interpretation difficult. This pattern must not be confused with that associated with bacterial infection, but if smears are repeatedly unsatisfactory in this group of women, colposcopy may be the only reliable means of excluding cervical intraepithelial neoplasia.

Some areas of real difficulty remain, as in the case of women with smears showing large numbers of keratinized squamous cells and little else. The cells are often anucleate. These appearances suggest extensive leucoplakia; it is impossible to assess any change that may be occurring in the cells beneath the surface and thus predict the underlying pathology. One repeat smear after three months may be appropriate, with referral for colposcopy if a similar pattern is seen. However, where the facility exists, immediate referral should be considered.

Atypical glandular changes, not sufficiently marked to warrant a diagnosis of adenocarcinoma, may be very difficult to manage cytologically. Discus-

Table 4.1 Cytological indications for referral for colposcopy

1 Suggestion of invasive carcinoma
2 Severe dyskaryosis
3 Moderate dyskaryosis
4 Persistent mild dyskaryosis/borderline nuclear changes
5 Persistent unsatisfactory smears
6 Suggestion of glandular lesion
7 Excessive numbers of keratinized cells

sion with the clinician and colposcopist over individual cases is a sensible approach (see Chapter 11).

OTHER REASONS FOR REFERRAL

Reasons for referral other than an abnormal cervical smear should not be overlooked. A woman who has a clinically 'suspicious looking' cervix to naked eye examination, in spite of whether or not the cervical smear is reported as showing dyskaryotic or malignant cells, should be referred for colposcopy.

It is often claimed that the diagnosis of invasive cancer of the cervix is a clinical one, but, as many general practitioners and clinicians may not see a case of invasive disease in their professional lifetime, early invasive disease can easily be missed. Many women with cervical cancer suffer from intermenstrual and postcoital bleeding, and therefore in such cases colposcopy may be of benefit.

When areas of leucoplakia (hyperkeratinization) can be seen at speculum examination, referral for colposcopy and biopsy ought to be considered, as the layers of keratin mask the true nature of the underlying epithelium from the cytologist.

It is clear that women with vulval and vaginal intraepithelial neoplasia, as well as those with vulvovaginal warts, are at increased risk for cervical intraepithelial neoplasia. This group should also have priority in a protocol for referral for colposcopy, even if the cervical smear is negative.

5. Taking a Screening Smear

INTRODUCTION

There are aspects which are of special significance as regards the actual taking of a cervical smear, and those will be discussed here. Other considerations relating to the ambience of the clinic, its facilities and the comfort of women being colposcoped, are discussed in detail in Chapter 21.

VISUALIZATION OF THE CERVIX

The first essential prerequisite is that the entire cervix must be fully visualized, and a speculum of suitable size should be chosen. In a well woman, prior manual examination is not acceptable, because, if a lubricant is used or bleeding is instigated, the smear will become contaminated and rendered unsatisfactory for assessment. Whether the speculum is warmed under running tap water before insertion is a matter of preference. As a rule, lubrication is best avoided, but if it is not possible to manage without it, then it should be used sparingly and not be allowed to come in contact with the cervix.

Whether the left lateral or lithotomy position is used (Fig. 5.1) is a matter of personal preference, but there should be a source of good illumination and the cervix should be completely and clearly visible.

TYPE OF SPATULA

For many years, the only type of cervical spatula available was the Ayre's design. It has become increasingly clear that no one instrument is ideal in all cases. Currently, there are numerous varieties of cervical sampling devices available; it is recommended that a selection of samplers be available on the clinic trolley, and that some thought is given to selecting the optimal device for various situations (Fig. 5.2).

The Aylesbury spatula is a modified Ayre's spatula in wood with an elongated and thinner prong, and in the vast majority of women it will be the optimal type. Several commercial variants of this design, both in wood and in plastic, are available (Fig. 5.3), but some are relatively expensive. The thinner extended prong allows more effective sampling of the endocervical canal, with a higher yield of endocervical glandular cells at the same time as sampling the ectocervix with the broad part of the blade of the spatula, thus increasing confidence that a truly representative sample has been obtained.

In the case of a large, patulous or multiparous cervix, a broader spread is most suitable, still taking care to sample the endocervical canal. This requires thorough scraping of the ectocervix over the whole area, using the broad, flat end of the spatula in a backwards and forwards movement which is more akin to painting.

At the other end of the spectrum, a small, tight postmenopausal or postconization os, with no visible transformation zone, demands careful sampling of the canal. On occasions, even the thin prong of an Aylesbury spatula will be too large to sample the target area effectively, and a suitable alternative could be the endocervical brush. It must be emphasized that, apart from the instances where there has been previous colposcopic assessment, the endocervical brush should not be used routinely on its own. Problems associated with it include bleeding from the canal, and sometimes damage of epithelium in a visible squamocolumnar junction.

Ideally, the endocervical brush should be used in combination with an Aylesbury or similar type of spatula. The usually employed method is to use each

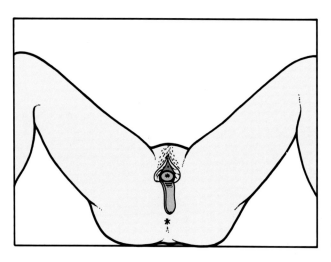

Fig. 5.1 Diagrammatic representation of the lithotomy position. The cervix is visualized by inserting a speculum (not shown) for taking a cervical smear.

Fig. 5.2 Selection of commercially available sampling devices. (a) Aylesbury; **(b)** Histolab; **(c)** Medscand; **(d)** Ayre's.

Fig. 5.3 Modifications of Ayre's spatula.

consecutively, inserting the spatula first, smearing it on a slide, taking a specimen with the brush and smearing that on the slide (Fig. 5.4). Speed is important, to prevent the material smeared from the spatula becoming air dried before the brush material is smeared. The use of two slides would overcome this problem, but would increase the work for the cytology laboratory. Another alternative is to use the spatula and brush together, leaving the brush in the canal while the spatula is being rotated, withdrawing both at the same time and smearing them together on the same slide.

The device used will be a matter of preference based on experience and, to some extent, financial constraints. Perhaps the most difficult concept to grasp is that of variety, and learning to tailor the sampling device to suit a particular cervix, as opposed to the established tendency to use one universal sampler for all cervices.

a. spatula inserted in os and rotated

b. endocervical brush inserted in os and rotated

Fig. 5.4 Diagrammatic representation of obtaining a cervical smear, using (a) a spatula and (b) an endocervical brush.

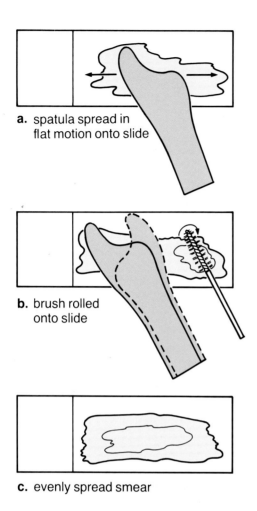

a. spatula spread in
   flat motion onto slide

b. brush rolled
   onto slide

c. evenly spread smear

Fig. 5.5 Diagrammatic representation of the optimal method of spreading a cervical smear.

SPREADING THE SMEAR AND FIXATION

The method of spreading the material on to a glass slide also needs to be carried out with care and thought. It is important to spread the material evenly, avoiding thick areas which would result in incomplete penetration of the fixative (Fig. 5.5); the latter would give rise to artefact (Fig. 5.6) or dense staining (Fig 5.7), making cytological assessment impossible.

The next critical step is fixation. If the sample is allowed to air dry at all, quality will be seriously impaired in terms of preservation of vital cell detail as well as staining, which may render the smear at best suboptimal and at worst unsatisfactory for a reliable assessment (Fig. 5.8). Once spread evenly, and using

Fig. 5.6 Unsatisfactory smear: fixation artefact.
Numerous cells show a brown precipitate over the nuclei, which is the result of delayed fixation in this case. A similar appearance can be due to poor staining or mounting in the laboratory.

Fig. 5.7 Unsatisfactory smear: too thickly spread. The nuclear detail is quite impossible to assess in this thick clump of cells, and there is evidence of incomplete penetration of fixative and stain in the central area.

Fig. 5.8 Unsatisfactory smear: air drying. Delay before fixation has resulted in a bloated appearance to the cells, so that chromatin detail is lost, making interpretation difficult. The larger cells at the upper left edge of the central group are almost certainly dyskaryotic.

all the material obtained on the spatula, the slide must be either completely immersed in 95° alcohol, or flooded with polyethylene glycol fixative (Fig. 5.9). It is important to ensure that the fixative is fresh and not previously used, as cell fragments and debris are frequently lost and quickly contaminate fixative pots and dishes. The slides should be well separated and not touch one another, to allow free circulation and rapid penetration of fixative.

IDENTIFICATION AND LABELLING

Correct labelling of all smears is of prime importance. Frosted end slides should be used. On each slide there should be the surname of the woman, together with forename for more common surnames, clinic number or name, date, and type of specimen, for example, cervical or vaginal. A lead pencil should be used, since most inks are soluble in alcohol fixative. It is important that this information is written on the slide before the smear is taken, as vital seconds can be

lost and the smear rendered unsatisfactory if it is added after the smear has been spread.

Every smear should be accompanied by a completed request form, clearly filled in block capital letters to minimize incorrect interpretation (Table 5.1). Surname, forename, date of birth and relevant clinical data should be included, particularly if there is a history of intermenstrual or postcoital bleeding (see page 62). It is helpful to know if there is a history of a previous abnormal smear, or whether any treatment has been given, as follow up and recommendations may be dependent on the type and time of such treatment. A menstrual history, with the date of the last menstrual period, is important in all cases.

The cytologist should also be informed of any use of hormones, including oral contraception, if a proper assessment is to be achieved. It is necessary that information regarding the type of specimen is included, since cellular constituents will vary from one site to another; cell types may be quite acceptable in a cervical smear, but are of special significance in a vaginal smear. Recommendations for referral or

a. smear flooded immediately and completely with fixative (polyethylene glycol); should not be allowed to air dry

gloved hands

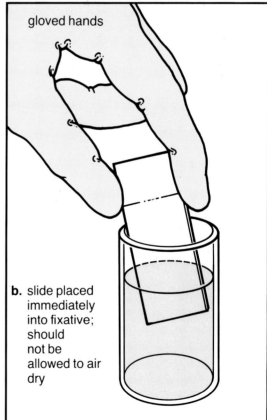

gloved hands

b. slide placed immediately into fixative; should not be allowed to air dry

Fig. 5.9 Diagrammatic representation of fixing a cervical smear. The slide is immersed in 95° alcohol, or flooded with polyethylene glycol.

Table 5.1 Information required on cytology request forms

Patient identification
Surname
Forename
Date of birth
Full postal address
Full postal address of family doctor

Clinical details
Type and source of smear (cervix, vulva, endocervical brush)
Relevant symptoms (e.g. intermenstrual bleeding, profuse discharge)
Details of any hormonal treatment or other medication
Date of last menstrual period
Previous history of abnormal smear with details of any treatment

Clinic details
Name of clinic or ward
Clinic or hospital registration number
Name of consultant
Name of taker of smear

All information should be clearly written, preferably in block capitals, in order to avoid misinterpretation. Additional information may be required for local reasons or as the result of national policies.

Table 5.2 Reasons for unsatisfactory smears

1 Faulty clinical procedures
Too scanty
Too thickly spread
Inadequate fixation
Incomplete visualization of cervix

2 Hormonal status
Menstrual
Excessive progesterone effect
Late secretory
Oral contraceptive

3 Cytological appearances
Red blood cells
White blood cells
Bacteria
Unrepresentative sample

follow up may be inappropriate if misleading information is given.

It is now mandatory for a woman as well as her physician to be informed of the result of any cervical smear, and therefore the full postal addresses of both are necessary.

UNSATISFACTORY SMEARS

Table 5.2 summarizes the reasons for unsatisfactory smears. Those relating to faulty clinical technique have already been discussed, and can be improved by proper training (see above). Similarly, the cytological decisions regarding the suitability of smears for a reliable assessment can be improved by an awareness of the areas of difficulty and application of quality assurance, both within the laboratory and by involvement in external systems. A balance has to be kept between smears that need to be repeated, and those which are satisfactory.

Unsatisfactory smears due to physiological reasons can be minimized by screening, as far as possible, between the tenth and the sixteenth day of the menstrual cycle. This should definitely be arranged for women having cervical smears as part of the call/recall programme. For diagnostic purposes, arrangements cannot always be convenient in this respect.

Whilst a menstrual smear, or a smear taken in the late secretory phase, are not inevitably unsuitable, it should not be a surprise if the report is classified as 'unsatisfactory'; it must be accepted that a proportion of smears will be justifiably reported as such, and a repeat smear will be required.

The question of absence of endocervical glandular cells in cervical smears is hotly debated, and opinions differ. In the United States, the view of the National Institutes of Health is that a cervical smear without endocervical glandular cells should be regarded at least as suboptimal. Some authorities are suggesting that such a smear should be reported as unsatisfactory.

However, the British Society for Clinical Cytology, together with the British Society for Colposcopy and Cervical Pathology, have issued a statement suggesting a more reasoned approach. This does not overemphasize the absence of endocervical glandular cells in a cervical smear as a sufficient reason in itself to render a smear unsatisfactory. Other factors should also be taken into account, including the age and hormonal status of the woman.

With practice, the procedure to obtain an optimal cervical smear can be carried out with ease and in a few minutes. However, it is important not to become overconfident; a less than fastidious technique can compromise a woman being screened and undermine confidence in cytology. Furthermore, it could unfairly diminish the confidence of the cytologist.

6. Introduction to Colposcopy and Documentation

THE COLPOSCOPE

Introduction and historical background

The colposcope is a microscope designed to allow examination of the cervix with magnifications ranging between six- and 40-fold. It was invented by Hinselmann, and was first described by him in 1925. Hinselmann, like others in his time, felt the need to diagnose cancer of the cervix in its earliest possible form, and thought that if the cervix could be magnified with the use of an optical instrument, cancer would become visible at its earliest stage, either as a small ulcer or a small exophytic lesion. Hinselmann soon realized that his suppositions were incorrect, but nevertheless found it possible to see changes in the cervical epithelium which fell outside the limits of normality.

In the early days, the technique of colposcopy was confined to German speaking countries, and it was not until the 1960s that the English speaking nations began to take an interest in it. Although its lack of popularity outside Germany was, to some extent, due to the fact that the original work was published in German, it was further hampered by an impression that its only value was as a research instrument. While accepting the value of the colposcope in research, its main function is, undoubtedly, purely clinical.

When Hinselmann first came across cervical cytology, his reaction was that this method would mean the end of colposcopy. However, after seeing and assessing cytology, he realized that the two techniques were complementary, and stated that "the man who thinks that cytology is better than colposcopy, or that colposcopy is better than cytology, is a fool who knows nothing of either."

At this point, the place of histology should be stressed: while it is important that the colposcopist is aware of the terminology used by the cytologist, it is even more important that the colposcopist has a working knowledge of the histology of normal and abnormal cervix, and is fully familiar with the terminology used by the histopathologist.

Types of colposcope

Several types of colposcope have been produced, but all are based on the principles of magnification, usually ranging between six- and 40-fold, and adequate illumination in order to visualize the cervix. Modern light sources usually rely either on a tungsten or halogen lamp, or a fibreoptic cable.

The colposcope is usually mounted on a freely moveable stand. Alternatively, it can be fixed to the side of an examination table, or be attached to a wall or the ceiling of the colposcopy room (Fig. 6.1).

The focal length of the colposcope usually ranges between 200 and 250 mm, which is a comfortable working distance for most practitioners. However, some colposcopists, like Kolstad, use an objective lens of 125 mm, while others use lenses of up to 400 mm. The longer working distance may be preferable when operative procedures are being carried out under colposcopic direction. There are varying magnifications for eyepiece lenses, ranging between six- and 12-fold, and drum changers for large magnifications.

Most colposcopes have various accessories, such as:

1. A monocular teaching arm.
2. A still or video camera (the latter has largely superceded 1).
3. A green filter which is interposed between the light source and the objective lens of the colposcope. The green filter absorbs red light, so that red blood vessels become much darker and appear black. The green filter is a particularly important accessory if the saline technique is being practised for colposcopy.

Fig. 6.1 Modern video documentation. A tiny, unobtrusive, colour video camera (actual size: 2 × 2 × 2 inches) is attached via a beamsplitter between the colposcope body and eyepiece section. Courtesy of Karl Zeiss, Germany.

TECHNIQUE OF COLPOSCOPIC EXAMINATION

Instrumentation

THE EXAMINATION TABLE

Any form of examination table which allows the patient to be placed in a modified lithotomy position is suitable for colposcopic examination. The patient's feet can be placed either in heel rests or in knee crutches (Fig. 6.2).

It is not essential to have a chair which can be moved up or down (see Fig. 6.2), although this has an advantage, particularly where operative procedures are being carried out under colposcopic direction.

A typical range of instruments is shown in Fig. 6.3. Those are placed on the trolley situated alongside the colposcopist. The following instruments are essential:

1. Bivalve speculum (Fig. 6.4). Varying widths of specula should be available, and the colposcopist should be encouraged to use the widest size which can be most comfortably inserted into the vagina. Routine use of a narrow speculum is to be discouraged, as visualization of the cervix will often be restricted by lax vaginal walls.
2. Cotton wool balls.
3. Sponge-holding forceps, to hold the cotton wool balls.
4. Cotton swabs or orange sticks with a tip covered in cotton wool.

Fig. 6.2 Colposcopy couch with knee rests. This can be moved up and down, and will tilt. Courtesy of Rocket of London.

Fig. 6.3 Colposcopy instrument trolley.

Fig. 6.4 Cusco speculum. (a) Bivalve. **(b)** With smoke extractor attachment: this is necessary for laser and diathermy treatment.

5. Endocervical speculum, useful for examining the endocervical canal (Figs 6.5 and 6.6).
6. Iris hooks. These are used by ophthalmologists and are very useful in colposcopy, as the very fine hook can be inserted into the cervical or vaginal epithelium with minimal or no discomfort, thereby allowing manipulation of the cervix or vagina under direct vision (Fig. 6.7). The hook is usually detachable, and the length of the handle can be adjusted to suit individual needs. Alternatively, a skin hook may be used, which has a larger hook than the iris type.
7. Biopsy forceps (Fig. 6.8), several types of which are available. A number of them are purpose-made, but some colposcopists use bronchoscopy or sigmoidoscopy biopsy forceps.
8. Four small containers. These hold normal saline solution, acetic acid (3% or 5%), Schiller's iodine (iodine 2 g, potassium iodide 4 g and distilled water 300 ml) and Monsel's solution.
9. Endocervical curette.

Examination procedures

The patient is placed in a modified lithotomy position, and the cervix is exposed using a bivalve speculum. There are two basic schools of colposcopy: that which practises 'classical or extended' colposcopy, and that which uses the 'saline technique'.

CLASSICAL OR EXTENDED COLPOSCOPY

This is the method most widely used. The cervix and upper vagina are first examined at six- to 16-fold magnifications. If a cervical smear is thought necessary, it should be obtained at this stage, taking care not to scrape the cervix too vigorously; otherwise bleeding may occur, causing difficulties in interpreting the subsequent colposcopic picture.

Following this, excess mucus is gently removed from the cervix with a dry or saline soaked cotton wool swab. Again, the cervix is inspected. Routine

Fig. 6.5 (a) Kogan's endocervical speculum. (b) Magnified view of the distal end.

Fig. 6.6 Visualization following insertion of endocervical speculum. (a) Acetowhite epithelium is seen extending into the endocervical canal. **(b)** The endocervical speculum allows the upper limit of the lesion to be very clearly seen.

smear taking at the first visit is not always necessary, as usually the colposcopist will already know that the cytology is abnormal.

Acetic acid test

Acetic acid (3% or 5%) is gently applied with a cotton wool swab. Acetic acid is left in situ for approximately five seconds; it is then relatively easy to remove most of any remaining mucus. The acetic acid causes the tissue to swell, especially columnar and abnormal epithelium; the latter appears as white epithelium (acetowhite), which is usually quite easily distinguishable from normal epithelium because of a sharp line of demarcation between the two. Normal squamous epithelium appears pink, as colposcopic illumination picks up the redness of the subepithelial capillary pattern.

As the effect of acetic acid depends on the amount of nuclear protein present, it follows that abnormal epithelium, because of its higher nuclear density and consequently higher concentration of protein, will undergo maximal coagulation and prevent light from passing through the epithelium. As a result, the subepithelial vessel pattern is less easy to see, and therefore the epithelium appears white. The higher the concentration of protein, the more intense the white appearance will be, following application of acetic acid.

The acetic acid effect wears off after approximately 30–40 seconds, but reappears if application is repeated. Following application of acetic acid, Schiller's iodine may be used.

Schiller's iodine test

The rationale behind this test is that normal, mature, squamous epithelium is characterized by an abundance of glycogen, whereas abnormal epithelium contains relatively little or no glycogen. Therefore, application of Schiller's solution to normal squamous epithelial cells will produce a dark brown, almost black stain, whereas columnar and abnormal epithelial cells, both of which contain little or no glycogen, remain relatively unstained.

Most experienced colposcopists do not routinely use this test, although it is essential that beginner colposcopists use it, as occasionally minor degrees of abnormality will be recognized which would otherwise remain undetected.

Colposcopists should also remember that false positive Schiller's tests are relatively common. In particular, immature metaplasia and a congenital transformation zone will be non-staining. Sometimes, these conditions cover large areas of the cervix and may even extend on to the vagina; since they do not require treatment, it is important that they are recognized for what they are: variations of normal epithelium.

SALINE TECHNIQUE

The use of acetic acid or Schiller's iodine makes a study of the angioarchitecture of the cervix difficult. For this reason, the saline technique was devised by Koller and developed by Kolstad, both from the Norwegian Radium Hospital, in Oslo.

After the cervix is exposed, mucus is gently removed with a cotton wool swab and the cervix moistened with physiological saline; this allows the subepithelial angioarchitecture to be studied in great detail. In order to see capillaries most clearly, it is advisable to use a green filter at high magnification; the red capillaries will appear darker and stand out more clearly.

This method depends entirely on the visualization

Fig. 6.7 Iris hook.

Fig. 6.8 Tips of three commonly used cervical punch biopsy forceps.

of various vessel patterns, and although it is a more difficult technique to master, it allows the colposcopist to predict the underlying histological pattern with greater accuracy than the acetic acid method.

COLPOSCOPIC BIOPSY

If the colposcopist contemplates treatment of cervical intraepithelial neoplasia by destruction (cryocautery, cold coagulation, deep radical diathermy or laser), it is imperative that a colposcopically directed biopsy is taken and assessed by an expert pathologist before such treatment is undertaken (Fig. 6.9).

However, if the patient is to be treated by cone biopsy, there is little point in taking an outpatient biopsy unless there is suspicion of invasion. Several forceps are available, all of the punch biopsy type.

The biopsy site must be chosen with care, and should be that part of the cervix which shows the greatest degree of abnormality. If necessary, several biopsies should be taken. Occasionally, the biopsy forceps may slip off the ectocervix, in which case the epithelium can be raised by using an iris hook or, alternatively, a single toothed tenaculum. Bleeding can be arrested quite simply with a silver nitrate stick or Monsel's solution (Table 6.1 and Fig. 6.9c).

For best haemostatic results, Monsel's solution should be used as a paste. This is produced by leaving a small amount (10–20 ml) of the solution in a small, open container for 24–72 hours. If the paste solidifies through being exposed for a longer time, a little of the original solution may be added and stirred until the paste-like consistency is restored. The paste is applied directly to the biopsy site using a small cotton wool tipped stick.

Cartier has described the method of taking cervical biopsies using a diathermy loop. This technique has now been adapted to allow removal of the entire transformation zone in the outpatient department, if desired, using a large diathermy loop (see Chapter 13, page 151).

A biopsy from the endocervical canal may be obtained with an endocervical curette. This technique is performed routinely in most North American centres; the aim is to detect unsuspected abnormality in the endocervical canal above the squamocolumnar junction.

A routine endocervical curettage may be helpful in preventing litigation, if the colposcopist admits to being relatively inexperienced. However, most experienced colposcopists reserve endocervical curettage for patients who have been treated by destruction or conization, and in whom the squamocolumnar junction is not visible; a sample is taken from the endocervical canal, to confirm that treatment has removed the entire epithelial abnormality. Alternatively, an endocervical brush may be used for obtaining a cytological sample from the canal (see page 51).

PSYCHOLOGICAL EFFECTS OF COLPOSCOPIC EXAMINATION

To be told that a cervical smear is abnormal and that colposcopy, and probably treatment, is required, may be a devastating experience for a woman. The utmost care must be taken to deal with the patient in a sensitive and understanding manner, with full awareness of her distress and fear. The patient should be carefully counselled when first told of her abnormal smear, and again before and after the colposcopic assessment; time for this should be available during her visit to the clinic.

As the cervical smear is usually thought of as a 'cancer test', many women with abnormal results will believe that they have cancer unless it is explained to them that they do not. During the examination, it

Fig. 6.9 (a) A cervical punch biopsy. (b) Immediately after punch biopsy. **(c)** After application of Monsel's solution for haemostasis.

Table 6.1 Monsel's solution (ferric subsulphate solution) (20 × 100ml)

Ferrous sulphate BP   – 2100 g
Nitric acid BP   – 150 ml
Sulphuric acid BP   – 110 ml
Freshly distilled water   – up to 2 litres
Nitric acid BP   – qs (sufficient amount)

- This product is to be prepared in the NSM fume cupboard as toxic fumes are given off (nitrogen dioxide). Fume cupboard fan to be on MAXIMUM and doors to weighing room kept ajar (to maximize ventilation).
- The operator must wear protective gloves, face mask and apron.
- Concentrated acids must be handled with extreme care and the equipment cleaned with care.

Method
DO NOT ALLOW VOLUME TO GO BELOW 2250 ml—STIR CONSTANTLY WITH MAGNETIC STIRRER.

1 Place 500 ml distilled water in a 5 litre beaker (previously tarred to 2 litres).
2 Measure out sulphuric acid. Have checked. Add it to the beaker.
3 Place the beaker on a hot plate/stirrer and heat to almost boiling.
4 Measure out 150 ml nitric acid. Have checked. Add it to solution in the flask.
5 Turn hot plate down to a low heat. Weigh out ferrous sulphate and have it checked. Gradually add it to the acid mixture with constant stirring: wait until it has dissolved and the effervescence has stopped before adding more. (Do not allow a sediment to form on the bottom.) Make up to 2250 ml approx. Bring to the boil.
6 Keep simmering gently on a medium heat. Gradually add approximately 40 ml nitric acid, then add dropwise until the red brown fumes stop evolving and the solution is a deep red colour. This usually needs about 70 ml. Watch for the red colour developing using a glass pipette to view the drops. Keep the volume between 2250 ml and 2500 ml.
7 Ask *Quality Control* to check that the solution is free from nitrate and ferrous ions. If not free of nitrates then boil it until it is. If ferrous ions are present not enough nitric acid has been added—repeat steps 6 to 8.
8 Aim to get the volume of solution to 2250 ml then allow it to cool.
9 Check the volume of the solution at room temperature in a measuring flask— make up to the volume with distilled water if below 2 litres.
10 Store in 100 ml brown glass bottles, and label. 30 ml are required for *Quality Control*.

Specimen label

NOT TO BE TAKEN   100ml
<u>FERRIC SUBSULPHATE SOLUTION</u>
(Monsel's solution)
DO NOT STORE BELOW 22 degrees C.
If exposed to low temperatures crystals may form which will redissolve on warming and shaking vigorously. Loosen cap before exposing bottle to heat.
KEEP OUT OF REACH OF CHILDREN
USE BEFORE: ....

needs to be made clear to the patient that she is the most important person in the colposcopy room. This is difficult to achieve in a teaching and research environment, but it is essential that observers are kept to a minimum. It is a good rule to allow only one observer, in addition to the colposcopist and nurse, with the patient's consent. Some clinics use suitable background music to good effect.

A colposcopic examination can be an unpleasant experience for a woman, but with sufficient thought and care by the clinic staff the psychological effects can be minimized.

DOCUMENTATION

History of the patient

Documentation of the patient's history may be performed using some modification of a standard gynaecological record layout, a specifically designed colposcopy page for insertion in the standard case records, a punchcard layout, or a specially designed software run on a microcomputer.

Obviously, personal preferences and financial considerations tend to dictate the choice, together with the caseload of the doctor or clinic. Also, the need to undertake intermittent clinical, research or other audit would influence the choice of a simple punchcard system, or, if it can be afforded, a computerized colposcopy patient record and management system.

STANDARD GYNAECOLOGICAL PAGE

This is the usual initial choice for the newcomer to colposcopy, involving no startup expense and allowing total personalization of the history record. However, there are clear disadvantages in assessing clinical and other outcomes, especially if the caseload becomes substantial.

Furthermore, this approach lacks the advantages of aide memoire, offered by other methods as a consequence of their systematized approach to direct questions in a patient's history.

SPECIFICALLY DESIGNED COLPOSCOPY PAGE

In addition to standard questions relating to the general gynaecological and obstetric history, this page would include a number of systematized questions pertinent to the range of disorders met in diagnostic colposcopy (Fig. 6.10).

If such an individualized sheet is to be redesigned and printed, it would be worth adding to the artwork diagrammatic representations of the cervical, vaginal and vulval outlines, with the anal region included, in the form of 'blanks' for drawing in longhand the colposcopic findings (see below).

PUNCHCARD SYSTEM

This is similar to the above page, but printed on a punchcard format (Fig. 6.11). Each individual element of a patient's history occupies one allocated closed perforation and, if present in a given case, it is converted to an open perforation using a special punching device.

Other perforations are attributed to elements of colposcopic findings, biopsies taken, histopathological diagnosis, cytological results, treatment employed with appropriate details, and any information required for research purposes.

The example in Fig. 6.11 also allows for longhand graphic recording of the topography and nature of any atypia within the transformation zone.

This method of documentation, by the use of a long needle-like device passed through the unpunched perforations in a uniform stack of cards, allows simple sorting of the group into sets and subsets, and subsequent counting by hand. This facilitates clinical and research audit, and is of value provided that patient numbers do not become too great.

Beyond a certain critical mass, the punchcard method becomes laborious, and has a further disadvantage in that these cards have to be kept separate from the casefolder, which may not be acceptable to a hospital records officer. Wasteful duplication of documentation may result.

COMPUTERIZED RECORDS AND MANAGEMENT SYSTEMS

Suitable software is currently becoming available for integrating computerized records and management of colposcopy patients. Such programs should offer a complete record of all aspects of a case (Fig. 6.12), including full personal details of patients, indications for referral, history, general clinical findings, specific colposcopic findings, biopsy sites, cytological and histopathological reports, and reports of other tests carried out during a visit (for example, bacteriological, virological). Details of decisions in relation to management should be recordable, and treatment detailed.

Subsequent follow up observations must be catered for, and the ultimate fate of the patient on discharge documented. Computer generated, standard letters to referring doctors and others with an interest in the case should be possible, with secretarial efficiency in mind. These should be user-definable. Preferably, the system should be capable of interfacing with the local 'well woman' cervical cytology call and recall computer, the cytopathology and histopathology reports computer system, and the hospital patient administration system.

The software must be user-friendly and attractive to clinicians. It is an advantage if the system can print out a visit summary for inclusion in the case records as hard copy, signed by the clinician for legal purposes.

With this type of documentation comes the problem of confidentiality, and therefore appropriate data protection and access codes are essential. Furthermore, in a large and busy clinic it is important to avoid unnecessary duplication of effort and material.

REFERRAL VISIT

COLPOSCOPY CLINIC

EIM62

Visit No. ....
Pat. No. ....

Date ....
Name ....

Seen by ....
DoB ....

LMP ....
Consultant ....

Reason for referral:—
  1. Abnormal smears de novo
  2. Abnormal smears after previous
      treatment of CIN
  3. Abnormal smears after previous
      treatment of carcinoma
  4. Clinically suspicious cervix
  5. DES exposure
  6. Routine after treatment elsewhere
  7. Other (specify):—

No. of pregnancies:—
  Births ....
  Spont. abortions ....
  Induced abortions ....

Referring cytology:—
  1. Class 0
  2. Class 1
  3. Class 2
  4. Class 3
  5. Not done

Current contraception:—
  1. Comb. pill   6. Female sterilization
  2. Prog. only   7. Male sterilization
  3. Condom   8. None
  4. Diaphragm   9. Other (specify):—
  5. IUCD

Present gynae symptoms:—
  1. None   6. Pregnant
  2. Abnormal discharge 7. Infertile
  3. IMB   8. Vulvar warts
  4. PCB   9. Other (specify):—
  5. PMB

Duration of abnormality (mths) ....
Approx. no. abnormal smears ....

Coitarche ....
Number ....

Previous history CIN/Carcinoma:—
  1. None
  2. Cone
  3. Laser
  4. Cold Coagulator
  5. Cryocautery
  6. T. Hyst
  7. Wertheim
  8. Radiotherapy
  9. Other (specify):—

Menstrual cycle:— (e.g. Reg K = $\frac{5}{26}$ 28)
Menstrual flow:—
  1. Heavy
  2. Not heavy
Dysmenorrhoea:—
  1. None/slight
  2. Moderate
  3. Severe

Smoking in the past 12 mths:—
Approx. no. per day ....
Serious medical disease
  1. No
  2. Yes:—

Other gynae history:—
  1. None
  2. D & C for menstrual problems
  3. PID
  4. Cautery (erosion)
  5. T. Hyst (not CIN)
  6. Subtotal Hyst
  7. Amputn cervix (PFR)
  8. Tubal/ovarian surgery
  9. Other (specify):—

Any other information:—
  1. No
  2. Yes:— see over

Fig. 6.10 Specifically designed colposcopy referral visit record page, for history details of patients. Courtesy of Dr G Smart, Edinburgh.

Fig. 6.11 Specifically designed punchcard for documentation of colposcopy history and findings. Courtesy of Dr I D Duncan, Dundee.

Findings

On completion of a diagnostic colposcopic examination, it is essential to document the findings, in the interests of good practice, for research purposes, and also for medicolegal reasons.

Documentation options include a simple longhand drawing, one of the variants of colpophotography, recording of a video image, and possibly the use of a microcomputer system with a sophisticated graphics element in the software.

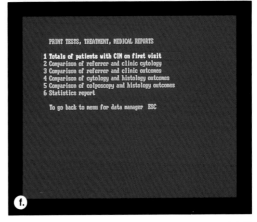

Fig. 6.12 Computerized colposcopy patient records and management system: examples of screens and documentation. (a) Patient identification and biodata. **(b)** Gynaecological and obstetric details. **(c)** Menu for operator.

(d) 'Failsafe' for patients without appointments. **(e)** Computer generated letter options. **(f)** Clinical audit statistical options. Courtesy of CTI Information, London.

COLPOSCOPIC ASSESSMENT

COLPOSCOPY CLINIC

EIM63

Visit No. ....

Date ....

Seen by ....

LMP ....

Pat. No. ....

Name ....

DoB ....

Consultant ....

Reason for examination:—
1. First visit
2. Routine post treatment
3. Abnormal cytology post treatment
4. Routine follow up
5. Other (specify):—

Appearances of vulva:—
1. Normal   4. Leucoplakia
2. Atrophic   5. Tumour
3. Warts   6. Other (specify):—

Appearances of vagina:—
1. Normal
2. Abnormal:—

Cervix:—
1. Present   2. Absent

Upper limited of TZ:—   Extent of TZ:—
1. Seen   1. <25%
2. Not seen   2. 25<50%
3. Equivocal   3. 50% +
                           4. −>vagina
                           5. none seen

Initial colposcopic appearance:—
1. Normal   6. Inflamed
2. Polyp   7. Atrophic
3. Condyloma   8. Malignant
4. Leucoplakia 9. Other (specify):—
5. Adenosis

Appearance with acetic acid:—
1. Normal   6. Coarse mosaic
2. Acetowhite 7. Microinvasive
3. Fine punctn 8. Invasive
4. Coarse punctn 9. Unsatisfactory
5. Fine mosaic

Schiller's test—extent of abnormal epithelium:—
1. <25%   4. −>vagina
2. 25<50%   5. none seen
3. 50% +   6. test not done

Endocervical curettage
1. Not done
2. No curettings
3. Tissues obtained

Biopsy taken: 1. No
                  2. Frozen Section
                  3. Paraffin
                  4. Both

Bx (0'C)

Histology

Smear taken:—
1. No   Ref. No. ....
2. Yes

Photograph taken:—
1. No   Ref. No. ....
2. Yes:—

PV findings:—
1. Normal
2. Significant uterine enlargement
3. Clinical cervical carcinoma
4. Cervical excitation pain
5. Adnexal mass(es)
6. Pregnant
7. Not done
8. Other (specify):—

MANAGEMENT AND DISPOSAL:—
Please Complete Management / Return
Visit Sheet as appropriate.

Fig. 6.13 Specifically designed and printed colposcopy record page, with a facility to document findings for the cervix and upper vagina.
Courtesy of Dr G Smart, Edinburgh.

LONGHAND DRAWING

This is the simplest method of documenting colpo-scopic findings. Diagrams may be drawn on printed outlines of the cervix, vagina and vulva, as discussed above (Fig. 6.13), but if these are not available they must be drawn as part of the representation (Fig. 6.14). For the cervix, it is imperative that, as a minimum, some indication is given of the limits of the transformation zone. In addition, the position of the anatomical external os is indicated. If the new squamocolumnar junction lies out of sight within the canal, this should be shown. The colposcopist carefully draws in areas of abnormality, using a devised system of shading, cross-hatching, annotation, etc.

The system should cover glandular mucosa and gland openings, leucoplakia and acetowhite change, mosaic, punctation and atypical vascular patterns. Inflammatory vascular patterns, raised or uneven surface and micropapillary change should also be indicated.

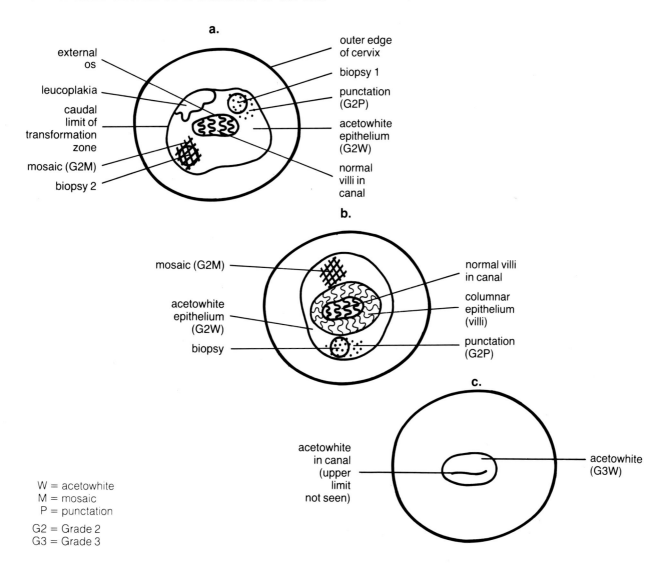

Fig. 6.14 Longhand drawing of the cervix. (a) This example represents a common distribution of abnormality. The transformation zone is totally ectocervical and composed mainly of acetowhite epithelium, with areas of punctation and mosaic. It is good practice to indicate the grade of abnormality on the labels of the diagram. An area of leucoplakia is also present. Normal, villous columnar epithelium in the canal is represented by parallel wavy lines, with confirmation in writing. The positions of the biopsy sites are shown by red circles. **(b)** In this example, normal endocervical tissue is present on the ectocervix and is represented by parallel wavy lines. Crescentic areas of acetowhite epithelium, showing mosaic anteriorly and punctation posteriorly, are present; biopsy is recorded from the posterior lip. **(c)** A small area of acetowhite epithelium is present on the ectocervix and passes into the canal; this is shown by an absence of the pattern that indicates columnar epithelium, with confirmation in the written label.

For cervicovaginal lesions, the findings may be represented as in Figs 6.15 and 6.16, and for the vulva as in Fig. 6.17. Also, in the vulval diagram, hairbearing skin should be shown, especially if this is a site of suspected intraepithelial neoplasia.

Some indication should be given of the correlation of findings following Schiller's test and those on colposcopy, particularly after application of acetic acid. Finally, the diagram should highlight the sites of any punch or other biopsies taken.

Colpophotography

The use of colour photography offers the ultimate in accuracy of representation, but it may be considered excessive for routine documentation. Regardless, it is essential as teaching material, and an important research tool.

Photographs are probably the most accurate way of comparing colposcopic images at intervals of time. This may be of some importance in circumstances where a given lesion is kept under surveillance over a period without treatment.

With colour, it is usual to employ a 35 mm format, which can also be used as lecture or teaching material. Polaroid colour cameras (Fig. 6.18) are also available and offer the advantage of an instant image, ensuring that the intended field and exposure have

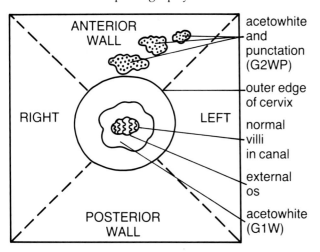

Fig. 6.15 Longhand drawing of the vagina. If the cervix is still present, it can be represented in the central part of the diagram. The anterior, posterior, left and right segments of the vaginal wall are identified diagrammatically, so that the location of the lesions can be recorded.

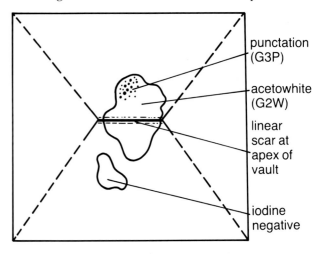

Fig. 6.16 Longhand drawing of the vagina posthysterectomy. In the absence of the cervix, the linear scars at the apex of the vault act as the central landmark. In other respects, the diagrammatic representation is similar to that shown in Fig. 6.15.

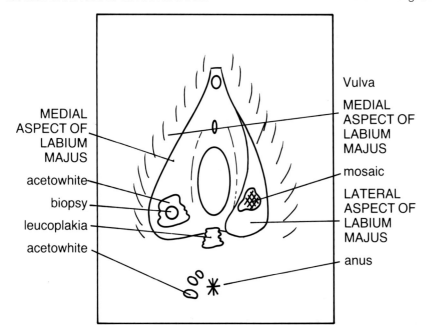

Fig. 6.17 Longhand drawing of the vulva. This should identify the exact position of the lesions so that the labia majora, both surfaces of labia minora, vestibule, fourchette and perianal region are represented.

been obtained. The instant print can also be annotated immediately and affixed to the patient's records.

Several special attachments are required to mount the camera on to the colposcope: a beamsplitter, which is inserted between the main colposcope body and binocular eyepiece; an adapter to connect the beamsplitter to the camera body (Fig. 6.19); a flash unit (Fig. 6.20) attached near or around the objective lens of the colposcope.

Closed circuit television

Using a similar arrangement, with a beamsplitter and a special C-mount adapter, a video colour television camera may be attached to record part of or the entire colposcopic examination (Fig. 6.21). This is used as a 'realtime' display, or as archives for teaching purposes.

Video could be used in routine documentation, although this is uncommon. In the future, the video medium may find a place if video laser disk technology for documentation becomes available. At present, it should be noted that apparatus is available which allows a virtually instant colour print to be produced from an image 'frozen' in a video frame. This process is less expensive per print than polaroid.

Fig. 6.18 Polaroid camera attached to colposcope via a beamsplitter and adapter.

Fig. 6.19 Special attachments for 35 mm colpophotography (beamsplitter and adapters).

Fig. 6.20 Flash unit, attached below objective lens on a colposcope body.

Fig. 6.21 Video camera attached to colposcope via a beamsplitter and C-mount adapter.

7. Colposcopic Appearances of the Normal Cervix

INTRODUCTION

There is a great deal more to colposcopy than simply the recognition of acetowhite epithelium, or epithelium which is non-staining after application of Schiller's iodine. The colposcopist must be aware of the following, easily observable, characteristic features of normal and abnormal cervical epithelium, as described by Kolstad:

1. Vascular pattern.
2. Intercapillary distance.
3. Colour tone relative to the junction of normal and abnormal tissue.
4. Surface contour.
5. Sharp line of demarcation between different types of epithelium.

ORIGINAL SQUAMOUS EPITHELIUM

The original squamous epithelium is easy to recognize, and with care four types of capillaries can be identified. These were first described in detail by Koller and Kolstad.

Hairpin capillaries

Terminal vessels of this type are characterized by one ascending and one descending branch of very fine calibre, forming a small loop. If the surface epithelium is not thick, it might be possible to observe the whole loop by colposcopy; generally, only the tip of the loop is visible, so that these hairpin capillaries are usually seen as regularly and densely arranged small dots (Fig. 7.1).

Fig. 7.1 Fine hairpin capillaries. The intercapillary distance varies between 50 and 200 µm.

Fig. 7.2 Fine network capillaries.

Fig. 7.3 Double hairpin capillaries, due to *Trichomonas vaginalis*.

Fig. 7.4 Branching vessels, seen in a normal transformation zone. Some are arranged around a gland opening (g).

Network capillaries

Occasionally, the terminal vessels of normal squamous epithelium are seen to form a dense, fairly irregular meshwork of very fine capillaries, referred to as network capillaries (Fig. 7.2).

Double capillaries

This term is applied to terminal capillaries of the hairpin type showing two or more crests at the top of the loop. Their shape may be described as resembling a fork, antler or clover leaf.

These latter loops are typically found in the presence of *Trichomonas vaginalis*, but can occasionally be seen within areas of cervical intraepithelial neoplasia (Fig. 7.3).

Branching vessels

These are larger, terminal vessels showing irregular branching patterns. The branches decrease stepwise in diameter, to terminate in a fine meshed capillary network. These vessels are confined to the transformation zone. They are particularly visible in the walls of retention cysts (Nabothian follicles), and around gland or cleft openings (Figs 7.4–7.6).

The inexperienced colposcopist may confuse these vessels with those of invasive carcinoma, but even with a little experience the two can easily be distinguished.

Original squamous epithelium is characterized by its typical, smooth, pink appearance (Fig. 7.7). If the surface is cleaned and moistened with saline, the typical hairpin-like capillaries will be recognized. Following application of acetic acid, the epithelium will still be pink, but the subepithelial capillaries will be more difficult to see. Whichever technique is used, there should be little difficulty in recognizing this epithelium.

Fig. 7.5 Branching vessels in a normal transformation zone.

Fig. 7.6 Branching vessels in a normal transformation zone.

Fig. 7.7 Normal pink squamous epithelium. The entrance to the endocervical canal is seen surrounded by columnar epithelium (centre). The junction of squamous and columnar epithelium is the squamocolumnar junction.

COLUMNAR EPITHELIUM

Normal columnar epithelium is easily recognized by its characteristic grape-like or villous appearance. Before application of acetic acid, the colposcopist will see that each columnar epithelial villus contains a fine capillary (Fig. 7.8). As the villus is covered by no more than a single layer of columnar cells, the blood in the capillary gives columnar epithelium its typically red appearance (Figs 7.9–7.12).

Following application of acetic acid, the villi often appear white and are more easily recognizable.

SQUAMOUS METAPLASIA

The transformation zone is the part of the cervix which is covered by mature normal squamous metaplasia, but which, at some point in the patient's life cycle, was covered by columnar epithelium. The new epithelium results from transformation of columnar to squamous epithelium, through the process of squamous metaplasia.

Mature metaplasia

Fully mature, squamous epithelium is characterized by the presence of gland openings and typical branching vessels, as described above (see Figs 7.4, 7.5 and 7.12). Nabothian follicles or retention cysts are also characteristic (Figs 7.13–7.15).

Immature metaplasia

Recognition of immature or active metaplasia, i.e. epithelium which is in the process of being transformed from columnar to squamous, is more difficult at this stage in the metaplastic process: the epithelium is acetowhite and can be very easily confused with abnormal epithelium. This situation may be

Fig. 7.8 Normal columnar epithelium. This shows capillaries in the villi; normal squamous epithelium; and the squamocolumnar junction.

Fig. 7.9 Columnar epithelium.

Fig. 7.10 Columnar epithelium.

Fig. 7.11 Cervix of a neonate. This shows normal columnar and squamous epithelium.

further complicated, because a cytological smear taken from immature metaplasia may not be reported as normal. Indeed, it is often difficult to differentiate between immature metaplasia and cervical intra-epithelial neoplasia (Figs 7.16 and 7.17).

Fig. 7.12 Normal transformation zone. This shows gland openings.

Fig. 7.13 Nabothian follicle.

Fig. 7.14 Multiple Nabothian follicles.

Fig. 7.15 Multiple Nabothian follicles.

Fig. 7.16 Immature metaplasia. (a) This 18 year-old woman presented with abnormal cervical cytology. **(b)** Colposcopy following application of acetic acid, showing acetowhite changes, punctation and mosaic capillary patterns. **(c)** Following application of Schiller's iodine, the epithelium is seen to be partially glycogenated. Histology confirmed immature metaplasia, with no cervical intraepithelial neoplasia. The woman was on combined oestrogen/progestogen contraceptive pills; the columnar epithelium in (b) shows enlargement and irregularity of the villi.

Coppleson and Reid described as follows the three stages of metaplasia which may be colposcopically recognizable (Fig. 7.18):

STAGE I

There is loss of translucency of the columnar epithelial villi, with each individual villus assuming a ground-glass appearance.

STAGE II

The grape-like configuration disappears as successive villi are fused and their intervening spaces filled in.

STAGE III

The villous configuration is lost, and the new surface takes on the appearance of a decreasingly translucent vascular area. Following fusion of the villi, the end result is normal squamous epithelium.

Scanning electron microscopy of metaplasia

The first stage of metaplasia is observed at the tips of columnar villi, where islands of larger metaplastic cells can be seen surrounded by normal columnar epithelium (Figs 7.19, 7.20). In the second stage, fusion of the columnar epithelial villi (Fig.7.21) can be seen with islands of flattened, irregularly polygonal cells surrounded by easily recognizable, smaller columnar cells.

In the first two stages of metaplasia, cells are covered with short microvilli, and there are no terminal bars between them. In the third stage of metaplasia terminal bars can be observed, similar to those seen between mature squamous epithelial cells, but the surface of these cells is still largely covered by short microvilli (Fig. 7.22).

When large areas of squamous metaplasia are examined at low magnification, its multifocal nature can be clearly seen. Cervical columnar epithelium

Fig. 7.17 Immature metaplasia. This 17 year-old woman presented with abnormal cervical cytology. The cervix is seen before **(a)** and after **(b)** application of acetic acid. The acetowhite epithelium was immature metaplasia.

Fig. 7.18 The three stages of metaplasia. See text for explanation.

Fig. 7.19 SEM of a columnar epithelial villus. Each villus is covered by columnar cells.

Fig. 7.20 Metaplasia, Stage I. Tips of a villus showing columnar (c) and metaplastic cells (m). SEM, × 2070.

often presents in a configuration of a series of ridges and clefts; if this is the case, it is the epithelium along the surface of the ridges which undergoes metaplasia first (Fig. 7.23).

Fig. 7.21 Metaplasia, Stage II. SEM of fusing villi.

Fig. 7.22 Metaplasia, Stage III. SEM showing flat, almost mature, squamous cells.

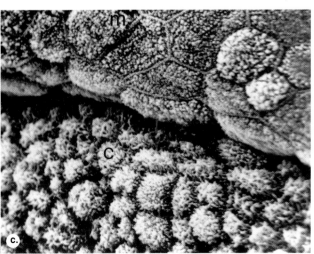

Fig. 7.23 Metaplasia. (a) Low power view of metaplasia (m) forming along the ridges, with columnar epithelium still present in the clefts. × 119. **(b)** Same area (m), showing the new squamocolumnar junction. × 477. **(c)** High power view of the same area, showing details of individual metaplastic (m) and columnar (c) cells.

CONGENITAL TRANSFORMATION ZONE

Whilst most areas of columnar epithelium undergoing squamous metaplasia reach full maturation into glycogenated squamous epithelium, showing the features described above, in a small number of patients metaplastic change results in a persistently acetowhite epithelium which is non-glycogenated. These changes are primarily confined to the cervix, but in approximately 4% of women this type of epithelium will extend from the cervix to involve the vagina, usually anteriorly and posteriorly (Figs 7.24–7.26).

This type of transformation zone may develop during intrauterine life, or prior to sexual activity, and is at no increased risk of neoplastic change. Its colposcopic significance is related to the following features: the epithelium is acetowhite, has a fine mosaic pattern (cf. cervical intraepithelial neoplasia), and is either non-glycogenated or partially glycogenated.

With histological confirmation of its benign nature no further treatment is required. However, the biopsy material is at risk of being misinterpreted, and the pathologist should be familiar with the typical histological appearances of this benign condition (Fig. 7.27). Therefore, if in the colposcopist's opinion such areas, which are usually very extensive, represent nothing more than a congenital transformation zone, the pathologist should be informed accordingly.

POSTMENOPAUSAL CERVIX

Following the cessation of oestrogen production, the squamous epithelium becomes atrophic with significantly fewer layers of cells. Because of this, one would expect the subepithelial capillaries to show through the thin epithelium, thereby giving the cervix a very red appearance. However, the underlying connective tissue is also changed, becoming less

Fig. 7.24 Congenital transformation zone, extending to the posterior vaginal wall. (a) Following application of acetic acid. **(b)** Following application of Schiller's iodine.

Fig. 7.25 Congenital transformation zone, extending to the anterior vaginal wall. (a) Before application of acetic acid. **(b)** Following application of acetic acid. **(c)** Following application of Schiller's iodine.

vascular; as a result the squamous epithelium looks pale and is hardly affected by application of acetic acid (Fig. 7.28).

Columnar epithelium becomes atrophic; the villi, characteristic of premenopausal columnar epithelium, become significantly smaller and in many instances disappear.

Application of Schiller's iodine also tends to stain the cervix and vagina a characteristic pale yellow. This is because there is lack of maturation of the squamous epithelium, which contains relatively little glycogen for staining with iodine. The endocervical mucus, characteristic of the premenopausal cervix, is now scanty and thick.

As the epithelium is very thin, insertion of a bivalve speculum may traumatize the small capillaries close to the surface, thereby producing subepithelial petechiae.

The postmenopausal cervix is often difficult for the inexperienced colposcopist to assess, particularly when the patient presents with an abnormal smear: often the squamocolumnar junction cannot be seen if it lies in the endocervical canal, which is a common postmenopausal feature. Under these circumstances, a short course of oestrogen will be very helpful: glycogenation increases, the mucus becomes clear, the cervix generally becomes softer, and an endocervical speculum can often be inserted to allow visualization of the squamocolumnar junction. Oestrogen may be administered as a cream or, alternatively, as an oral or transdermal preparation.

Fig. 7.26 Congenital transformation zone, associated with cervical intraepithelial neoplasia. This extends on to the anterior vaginal wall. Centrally, around the cervical os, there is an area of cervical intraepithelial neoplasia. In this case, provided the colposcopist can distinguish this from the congenital transformation zone, only the cervical intraepithelial neoplasia will require treatment.

Fig. 7.27 Congenital transformation zone; histology.

Fig. 7.28 Postmenopausal cervix. The epithelium is pale and atrophic, and subepithelial vessels can be seen. In some areas, there are subepithelial haemorrhages which have been caused by taking a cervical smear with a wooden spatula.

CERVICAL POLYPS

Cervical polyps almost invariably arise from endocervical columnar epithelium, and usually begin with the enlargement of a single epithelial villus. Their histological appearance is described in Chapter 1 (see page 7).

At its onset, the polyp is covered by columnar epithelium and may only be discovered during colposcopic assessment of the endocervical canal. As the polyp continues to grow, it will protrude beyond the external os. At this stage, metaplasia occurs: the tip of the polyp is covered first by immature and later by mature squamous epithelium, while the stalk, which usually remains in the endocervical canal, is covered by columnar epithelium (Figs 7.29 and 7.30).

The origin of the polyp, i.e. the point at which the stalk begins, must be determined, as removal of the tip but not the stalk will simply result in regrowth (Fig. 7.31). In order to identify the base of the stalk, the colposcopist must be aware that the polyp may not in fact arise from the endocervical canal; occasionally, endometrial polyps will present at the external os.

Less commonly, a submucous fibroid will develop a stalk and protrude through the endocervical canal, frequently causing irregular bleeding and appearing necrotic. Sometimes a necrotic polyp may lead to a false diagnosis of cervical carcinoma. The number of polyps should also be determined, as often more than one will be found. Malignancy in a cervical polyp is very uncommon but should always be considered.

Unless the base of the polyp is clearly visible and accessible, the endocervical canal should be assessed under general anaesthesia. The polyp and its stalk are removed, and the base of the stalk is treated by diathermy to prevent recurrence. Hysteroscopy will prove helpful where the base of the polyp is still not visible after dilatation of the cervix.

Fig. 7.29 Endocervical polyp. The stalk and base of the polyp are covered by columnar epithelium, whilst the tip is covered by squamous epithelium.

Fig. 7.30 Endocervical polyp. This is showing columnar and immature metaplastic epithelium.

Fig. 7.31 An endocervical polyp, arising in the endocervical canal. This is seen with the aid of an endocervical speculum.

8. Colposcopic Appearances of Cervical Intraepithelial Neoplasia

INTRODUCTION

With the saline technique, cervical intraepithelial neoplasia can be recognized: the abnormal epithelium is dark, there is a sharp line of demarcation between normal and abnormal epithelium, and the capillaries are readily visible, having a punctation or mosaic pattern or showing the presence of atypical vessels.

With the acetic acid technique, the abnormal epithelium appears white. There is a sharp line of demarcation between normal and abnormal epithelium, and the vessels, although less readily visible than with the saline technique, are much more visible than in normal epithelium. Occasionally, in minor degrees of cervical intraepithelial neoplasia there is no vessel pattern to be seen following the application of acetic acid – the abnormal epithelium simply appears white (Fig. 8.1).

Acetowhite change

Acetowhite change is the most important of all colposcopic features (see Fig. 8.1). All examples of cervical intraepithelial neoplasia, unless covered by keratin, will show some degree of acetowhiteness.

Table 8.1   Epithelial changes that may be acetowhite

Cervical intraepithelial neoplasia
Human papillomavirus infection
Combined CIN and HPV
Immature squamous metaplasia*
Healing/regenerating epithelium*
Congenital transformation zone
Inflammation*
Adenocarcinoma/adenocarinoma in situ*
Invasive squamous cell carcinoma*

* These conditions are often, but not invariably, acetowhite

Unfortunately, epithelial changes other than cervical intraepithelial neoplasia may also become white with acetic acid (Table 8.1), and it is important that these physiological and minor changes are recognized. Distinction by colposcopy alone is not always possible, and all abnormal areas should be biopsied.

Vascular pattern of abnormal epithelium

The vascular patterns associated with abnormal epithelium are as follows:

Fig. 8.1 Acetowhite change within the transformation zone. (a) No abnormal vascular pattern. **(b)** Similar, with gland openings and squamocolumnar junction clearly visible. **(c)** Same as (b), with more pronounced acetowhite change. **(d)** Very marked acetowhite change. CIN 3 was confirmed on biopsy.

PUNCTATION

This pattern is easily recognized, being characterized by dilated, elongated, often twisted and irregularly terminating vessels of the hairpin type, arranged in a prominent punctate configuration (Fig. 8.2). This is usually a well defined area so that there is a sharp line of demarcation between the normal and abnormal epithelium (Fig. 8.3). The dilated hairpin capillaries seen in inflammatory states (Fig. 8.4) should not be confused with punctation: when the capillaries are dilated and recognizable because of inflammation, the pattern is very diffuse, the capillaries are close together, and there is no sharp line of demarcation as would be seen between normal and abnormal epithelium.

Punctation vessels are more widely spaced than the hairpin capillaries seen in normal squamous epithelium, and because they extend closer to the surface they are more readily seen. Their shape may be hairpin-like, but occasionally they will resemble double capillaries, or the capillary loops may appear like a little ball.

MOSAIC

The capillaries are arranged parallel to the surface in a characteristic mosaic or 'crazy paving' pattern (Fig. 8.5). Therefore, vessels enclose a vascular field which may be small, large, round, regular or irregular in shape. Mosaic vessels may be fine and smoothly curved, coarse and irregularly curved, or they may consist of intertwining strands of dilating capillaries. However, whatever the fine structure, the overall

Fig. 8.2 Punctation. (a) Saline technique, before application of acetic acid. **(b)** After application of acetic acid. Note that the vascular pattern is now less pronounced.

Fig. 8.3 Punctation within a field of cervical intraepithelial neoplasia. The saline technique has been used. The abnormal epithelium appears dark, and punctation vessels can be clearly seen. There is a sharp line of demarcation between the normal (light) and abnormal (dark) epithelium. The capillaries on the left are more spaced, which is indicative of a higher degree of cervical intraepithelial neoplasia, compared with the epithelium on the right.

Fig. 8.4 Inflamed cervix. Widespread, uniform pattern of hairpin dilated capillaries. Compare this with Fig. 8.3.

pattern is characteristically mosaic and easily recognized.

ATYPICAL VESSELS

These are terminal vessels which are easily seen by the colposcopist (Fig. 8.6). Typically, they are irregular in size, shape, course and arrangement, and the intercapillary distance is significantly greater than that which is found in normal epithelium. There is no particular pattern, the vessels being arranged in a totally haphazard way.

Intercapillary distance

This is the distance between vessels or space encompassed by the mosaic vessels. In normal squamous epithelium, the maximal intercapillary distance of the hairpin and network capillaries varies, but is approximately 50–200 μm with an average of 100 μm. On the other hand, the maximal intercapillary distance increases as the lesion becomes more severe, i.e. in CIN 1 the average intercapillary distance may be 200 μm, whereas in CIN 3 the greatest intercapillary distance is often 450–500 μm

(see Figs 8.3 and 8.5b).

It is not necessary to measure the vessels, as in time the colposcopist will be able to tell immediately whether these are close together or widely spaced. If comparison is needed, then the vessels in a lesion should be compared with the vessels in the adjacent normal squamous epithelium.

Colour tone

Following application of saline, abnormal epithelium appears much darker than normal epithelium (see Figs 8.3 and 8.5a), whereas after application of acetic acid the abnormal epithelium appears very white (acetowhite epithelium; see Fig. 8.5b). In both cases, and particularly with acetic acid, an easily recognizable, sharp line of demarcation between normal and abnormal epithelium can be observed.

Surface contour

The surface of a lesion can be described as smooth and even, or irregular. For example, normal squamous epithelium has a smooth surface, while columnar epithelium is easily recognized by its

Fig. 8.5 Mosaic vascular pattern.
(a) Saline technique before application of acetic acid. Note the dusky colour tone. **(b)** Same as (a), following application of acetic acid. Note also the increased intercapillary distance, and the line of demarcation from normal epithelium. **(c)** Coarse mosaic with saline technique. **(d)** Coarse mosaic within a wide field of acetowhite change. Note the gland clefts and white gland openings.

typical grape-like or villous appearance. At the other extreme, invasive cancer is characterized by an uneven or often exophytic growth pattern (see Fig. 10.29, page 109).

Line of demarcation

The borderline or line of demarcation between normal and abnormal squamous epithelium is usually sharp, due to the change in colour which is present in the abnormal epithelium. In contrast, the line of demarcation between normal squamous epithelium and inflammatory lesions is more diffuse. Also, almost always a sharp line of demarcation will be seen between normal squamous and normal columnar epithelium (squamocolumnar junction), particularly after application of acetic acid.

Leucoplakia

Leucoplakia is seen less commonly on the cervix than acetowhite epithelium, and the vascular abnormalities are detailed above. Normal original or mature metaplastic squamous epithelium of the cervix does not have a layer of keratin on the surface, but in some circumstances keratosis occurs and leucoplakia is seen at colposcopy.

An area of leucoplakia is white before acetic acid is applied (Fig. 8.7), and does not change in colour after application. It is usually seen as one or more raised plaques which may coalesce as the area becomes larger (Fig. 8.8). The outline of the area is usually irregular. When keratosis is only slight, such as in the congenital transformation zone, all that may be observed is a waxy, non-wettable surface which is slightly white before acetic acid is applied but may become a little whiter after application.

Leucoplakia presents problems to the colposcopist when assessing the cervix, because its presence hides the diagnostic changes of the underlying epithelium (Fig. 8.9). Although fully developed leucoplakia on the cervix is usually associated with cervical intraepithelial neoplasia, it may be seen overlying otherwise completely normal epithelium, often outside the transformation zone, or an early invasive carcinoma. For this reason, the presence of more than a very small area of leucoplakia within the transformation zone must be an indication for considering of excision of the zone.

GRADING OF COLPOSCOPIC FINDINGS

It has already been pointed out that, in mosaic and punctation patterns, the intercapillary distance increases as the degree of histological abnormality in the epithelium becomes greater. Punctation and mosaic may be additionally graded on the basis of coarseness of vessels and regularity of their pattern: the more severe the underlying lesion, the coarser the vessels are likely to be and the more irregular the pattern, the extreme being the atypical vessels of early invasive disease.

Acetowhite epithelium may also be graded, primarily according to the degree of acetowhiteness that is reached at the maximum whiteness. Of secondary

Fig. 8.6 Highly atypical vessels within a small focal lesion in the transformation zone. Note the corkscrew and comma shaped vessels, and other bizarre forms.

Fig. 8.7 Multifocal waxy leucoplakia, seen within the transformation zone. No application of acetic acid.

Fig. 8.8 Coalescent leucoplakia on the cervix.

importance are the rapidity with which the lesion reaches its maximum degree of whiteness, the length of time that whiteness is retained, and the sharpness of the line of demarcation. Not only do severe abnormalities become whiter than minor lesions, but they tend to become white more quickly and retain their whiteness longer than the mild changes, the latter also usually having a less distinct outline. These features are summarized in Table 8.2.

Two further points need to be made about grading colposcopic abnormalities. First, there is difficulty in comparing different areas of the same cervix ·if mosaic and punctation as well as acetowhiteness are present. It is not always easy to determine whether a particular area of punctation represents a more severe abnormality than an adjacent area of acetowhite epithelium. This dilemma may be important in deciding from which area to take a directed biopsy. If in doubt, both areas should be sampled.

Secondly, it has to be emphasized that colposcopic grading is just that: a grading of the colposcopic

Table 8.2 Features assessed in colposcopic grading

Acetowhite epithelium
Maximum whiteness reached
Rapidity of development of maximum whiteness
Length of retention of whiteness
Sharpness of outline

Mosaic and punctation
Intercapillary distance
Coarseness of vessels
Regularity of pattern

features; it is not an assessment of the histological grade of the underlying lesion. With experience, it may often be possible for the colposcopist to predict with accuracy the degree of cervical intraepithelial neoplasia present; indeed, trying to guess the degree of abnormality is a useful exercise, as it increases the care with which the examination is carried out.

Fig. 8.9 (a) Cervical smear, showing a cluster of moderately dyskaryotic cells above and to the left. Note the smudgy, pink, anucleate, squamous cells. **(b)** Same cervix, showing extensive, dense, waxy leucoplakia. Careful inspection of the small area of visible underlying epithelium in the canal on the posterior lip reveals a clear mosaic pattern; **(c)** Appearance after Schiller's test. Note the biopsy site at the '6 o'clock' position. **(d)** Histopathology of the biopsy reveals cervical intraepithelial neoplasia, with dense, overlying hyperkeratosis.

However, colposcopy is not sufficiently sensitive to discriminate consistently and with certainty between the grades of cervical intraepithelial neoplasia, especially when comparing one woman with another. This is particularly true in the case of acetowhite epithelium, where features other than the degree of epithelial abnormality contribute to the acetowhiteness. For example, an area of CIN 3 in a woman of 60 years is usually quite thin, thinner than an area of CIN 1 in a woman of 25 years.

First and foremost, colposcopy defines the distribution of lesions; hopefully, early invasive lesions may also be identified (Table 8.3; see Chapter 10). In most cases, high grade lesions can be determined from minor lesions, and many examples of herpes papillomavirus infection, squamous metaplasia and congenital transformation zone can be correctly identified. However, the capabilities of the technique do not extend to a precise histological grading of cervical intraepithelial neoplasia, or a confident distinction between intraepithelial neoplasia and other causes of acetowhiteness.

A colposcopic report should identify the distribution of the abnormal areas with their colposcopic features and colposcopic grading. The grade of cervical intraepithelial neoplasia can only be added to the report when the histology of the biopsy is known.

Table 8.3 Colposcopic features suggestive of invasion

Atypical vessels
Irregular, raised nodular surface
Large, complex lesion
Wide intercapillary distance
Severe changes with canal involvement

Congenital transformation zone

The congenital transformation zone is confusing in terms of acetic acid application (see Figs 7.24–7.27), as it becomes acetowhite slowly but usually retains its whiteness for a long time. Thus, as the whiteness of a central area of cervical intraepithelial neoplasia is fading, it may still be increasing in a surrounding area of congenital transformation zone. Eventually, the congenital transformation zone may be considerably whiter in appearance than the significant cervical intraepithelial neoplasia adjacent to it, which could mislead the inexperienced colposcopist into biopsying the wrong area.

Despite the fact that CIN 3 in the older woman is more nuclear-rich, CIN 1 in the younger woman may be more acetowhite because of its greater thickness.

9. Handling Biopsy Specimens

INTRODUCTION

A number of different tissue specimen types originate in the colposcopy clinic. It is, therefore, useful for the colposcopist to be aware of the way biopsy specimens, obtained in the clinic or operating theatre, are dealt with in the laboratory, as this has a direct bearing on the handling of material at the time of taking a biopsy.

It is important that those engaged in colposcopy and the histological assessment of biopsy material are familiar with its proper handling. The specimens involved are: (a) punch biopsies (from the cervix, vagina and vulva); (b) wedge biopsies; (c) cone biopsies; (d) endocervical curettage specimens.

As a total hysterectomy may sometimes be carried out on women with cervical intraepithelial neoplasia and glandular abnormalities, it is also relevant to consider the examination of a hysterectomy specimen. However, details of handling a radical hysterectomy specimen are beyond the scope of this book.

FIXATION

On removal, all specimens are placed in a container with fixative, the purpose of which is to inactivate the cellular enzymes so that autodigestion of the tissue does not take place; furthermore, the tissue is preserved in the state that it was in at the time of fixation. A wide variety of agents are available as fixatives.

Formalin

The most widely used fixative is formalin (formol saline), a solution of formaldehyde in water, buffered so that it is isotonic with tissue. Formalin has a number of advantages as a general purpose fixative: it is easily available and inexpensive, and has probably the least toxicity, compared with other fixatives. Furthermore, histopathologists are familiar with the appearances of formalin-fixed tissues. However, for cervical histology, formalin is not ideal.

Bouin's fluid

This contains formalin, acetic acid and picric acid, and is preferred because of the greatly enhanced preservation of nuclear detail, compared with formalin.

The disadvantages of Bouin's fluid are that it is relatively expensive, picric acid is explosive if allowed to dry out, and its vapour is even more irritating than that of formalin. However, these disadvantages are outweighed by the superior quality of the final stained section. Virtually all histological material illustrated in this book has been fixed in Bouin's fluid.

Formol sublimate

This contains mercuric chloride, and also results in excellent histological fixation. However, because of the health risks associated with mercury-containing compounds, formol sublimate has been banned from most histology laboratories.

FIXATION TIME

Fixation time is finite, and the size of a biopsy specimen determines the length of time necessary for penetration of the fixative. A small punch biopsy will fix in Bouin's fluid in one or two hours, but even a fairly small cone biopsy should not be further processed until it has been left in fixative for at least six hours. Prolonged immersion in Bouin's fluid results in increasing hardening of tissue, which is another of its drawbacks.

PUNCH BIOPSY

Specimens obtained from the cervix, vagina or vulva, using any of the several types of punch biopsy forceps available, are handled in the same way. It is very important that these specimens are correctly dealt with, so that the maximum information can be obtained from them. The biopsy, if taken properly, will consist of an ellipse of epithelium approximately 5 mm in length, and in the cervical biopsy the underlying stroma will have a depth of 3–5 mm (Fig. 9.1a). Vaginal and vulval biopsies tend to have less underlying lamina propria and dermis, because of the different consistency of these elements.

Biopsies are immediately placed in Bouin's fluid. In addition to the other advantages over formalin, small specimens are easier to handle after fixation in Bouin's fluid, due to the yellow staining. Fixation results in curling of the specimen, so that epithelium is on the outer, convex surface and the stroma on the inside (Fig. 9.1b). This facilitates correct orientation. The use of filter paper, glass coverslips or even cucumber squares has been advocated, but none of these aids is necessary for proper orientation of a specimen.

The fixed, curled biopsy is transversely bisected, producing two approximately pyramidal shaped pieces (Fig. 9.1c). These are then embedded in wax with the flat, cut surface downwards (Fig. 9.1d), so that this surface is cut by the microtome. Each piece is cut at three levels, and thus a total of six levels are examined through the biopsy.

This number of sections should be adequate for most purposes, and therefore step-serial sectioning is not necessary. Routine staining is by haematoxylin and eosin; mucin stains are sometimes used when glandular abnormalities are suspected or found.

Biopsies smaller than the ideal size can be handled in the same way. Although the absence of underlying stroma can make orientation difficult, the combination of tissue curling in Bouin's fluid and sectioning at several levels nearly always means that at least one out of the six sections cuts the epithelium at right angles, enabling a diagnosis of the epithelial abnormality to be made.

Histopathological reporting

The histopathologist reporting on a colposcopic biopsy should, of course, indicate what degree of epithelial abnormality is present, and whether invasion is seen or not. It is good practice always to make a definite statement on whether there is evidence of invasion or not, as absence of evidence of invasion is a requirement that must be met before local destructive treatment of cervical intraepithelial neoplasia can be carried out. If there is no stroma, no comment can be made about invasion.

As the definition of microinvasive carcinoma requires that a cone biopsy or a larger specimen is examined, microinvasive carcinoma cannot be diagnosed on a punch biopsy; more precisely, it cannot be distinguished from stage Ib invasive carcinoma. A statement such as 'stromal invasion is present' should be used, usually without further qualification. This indicates that a further diagnostic procedure, normally a cone biopsy, is required. Nevertheless, it is sometimes possible to make a definitive diagnosis of stage Ib invasive carcinoma on a colposcopic biopsy, where the whole of a large biopsy is virtually replaced by invasive carcinoma.

WEDGE BIOPSIES

Wedge biopsies are not usually taken in the colposcopy clinic, and are required when invasive carcinoma is strongly suspected. These specimens are best fixed in Bouin's fluid and, if possible, orientated so that sectioning perpendicular to the surface is carried out.

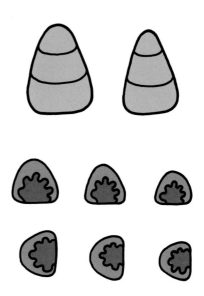

Fig. 9.1 Handling a punch biopsy specimen. (a) When freshly taken, the biopsy has a fairly flat layer of epithelium on the surface and stroma underneath. **(b)** After fixation in Bouin's fluid, the biopsy curls and the epithelium forms a rounded, convex surface. **(c)** The biopsy is transversely bisected. **(d)** Both halves are embedded in wax, with the cut surface facing down, and cut at three levels.

CONE BIOPSY

The term 'cone biopsy' describes the procedure of excising the transformation zone and producing a specimen suitable for histological examination. Excision may be carried out using a scalpel, laser (laser excision cone), or low voltage loop diathermy. The advantages and disadvantages of each of these methods are discussed in Chapter 13.

The specimens produced by all these methods are roughly similar and traditionally cone shaped, the base being the ectocervical surface and the apex the endocervical extreme. The current view is that the excised tissue should be cylindrical in shape, rather than conical, to avoid incomplete excision of the deeply involved endocervical crypts high in the canal. Because of the different emphasis in the indications allowing these procedures to be carried out in the outpatients department, laser excision cone specimens and low voltage loop diathermy specimens often tend to be shallower than knife cone biopsies. Therefore, it has been traditional for the surgeon to attach a stitch at one point of the circumference of the cone, to enable orientation. With the application of alternative methods, this practice seems generally to have been abandoned, and it is questionable whether knowledge of the exact position of the lesion in a biopsy is of any help in establishing future management. However, this knowledge is useful in correlating colposcopic findings with histological outcome.

Examination of cone biopsy specimens

A number of techniques have been proposed for the examination of cone biopsy specimens. To a certain extent, the method applied depends on the configuration of a specimen. Immediately upon removal, the specimen should be immersed intact into Bouin's fluid. It is common practice for the specimen to be opened, either by the gynaecologist or the pathologist; the cone is then pinned open and fixed. However, prior to fixation this will damage the fragile abnormal epithelium, and it is likely that the resultant stretching of the delicate endocervical epithelium significantly contributes to epithelial loss in the final sections. Opening of the cone biopsy specimen in no way facilitates examination of resection margins.

After fixation, most cone biopsy specimens can be dealt with in the same way (Fig. 9.2), by taking parallel cuts throughout the tissue. This must be done with a very sharp knife (such as a dermatome)

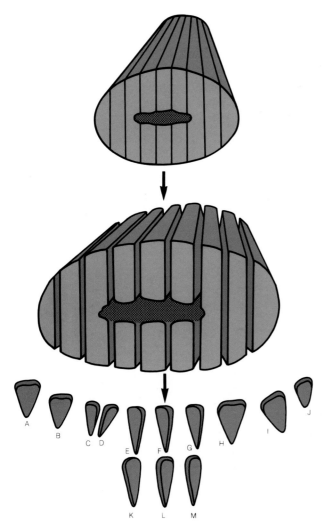

Fig. 9.2 Taking blocks from a cone biopsy. After thorough fixation in Bouin's fluid, the unopened specimen is divided into individual blocks of 2–2.5 mm thickness, each of which is initially sectioned at one level.

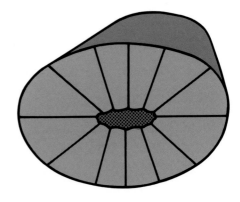

Fig. 9.3 Method of block taking when the cone has a wide open os.

at 2–2.5 mm intervals, taking care to keep the cuts straight and parallel (this is more easily achieved after fixation in Bouin's fluid than in formalin, because of the greater firmness of Bouin-fixed material). The corresponding surface of each block is sectioned (see Fig. 9.2), so that sampling is as even and thorough as possible. Oblique cuts are unlikely to be a problem with this technique.

Longitudinal sections are examined, and both ectocervical and endocervical edges of the specimen can be easily assessed.

It is unusual for the os to be circular and open. When it is, it may be necessary to take radial blocks (Fig. 9.3); this technique has the disadvantage that blocks end up being wedge-shaped, possibly causing a problem with embedding and sectioning. This approach is very rarely needed.

If the cone biopsy is long, an alternative approach can be used to good effect (Fig. 9.4). The endocervical part of the specimen is cut transversely, to obtain several circular blocks; if necessary, the block from the tip of the cone may be cut at levels, to assess the endocervical extreme. The ectocervical part of the cone biopsy is handled in the manner that has already been described, taking parallel anteroposterior cuts (see Fig. 9.4).

The cone biopsy specimen is sometimes not perfect and, perhaps as a result of distortion of the cervix, it may be open at one side. It is usually possible to handle this using a modification of the above methods (Fig. 9.5).

The techniques described above will generate approximately 6–25 sections, depending on the size of the cone biopsy. It is standard practice to examine, initially, just one good section from each block taken in this manner. If this first block shows anything suspicious, such as a focus of better differentiation within a gland crypt or an isolated focus of lymphocytic infiltration, both of which may indicate an adjacent area of invasion, deeper levels or step-serial sections are cut on that block, and usually also on adjacent blocks.

On the other hand, some centres advocate routine step-serial sectioning, resulting in perhaps 250 slides from the whole specimen. The policy of examining only one section from each block may be supported by the suggestion that, if an area of invasion is too small to be identified in sections taken at intervals of 2–2.5 mm, even if it was found by more meticulous sectioning, it is also too small to necessitate any change in the management of the patient.

Fig. 9.4 Method of block taking for a long cone biopsy. A transverse cut is made approximately 1.5 cm from the ectocervical edge, and serial transverse blocks are taken up to the endocervical end. The ectocervical part of the specimen is handled in the same way as the more usual cone biopsy. This method avoids the problem of unmanageably long blocks.

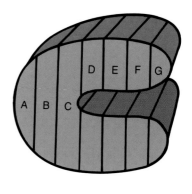

Fig. 9.5 Handling an opened cone biopsy specimen. The approach is basically the same as for a normal cone biopsy: the initial cuts are made at the joined end of the specimen.

THE CONE BIOPSY REPORT

The pathologist's report on a cone biopsy must give the following information:

1. The degree of cervical intraepithelial neoplasia, if any is present. It should also record whether crypts are involved or not, although this does not affect subsequent management. It will be helpful to the colposcopist if the distribution of the lesion (if the specimen can be orientated) and number of blocks involved by cervical intraepithelial neoplasia are indicated.

2. Whether invasion is present or not. The majority of specimens will not show invasion, but it is essential that a statement is included in the report making it clear to the gynaecologist that invasion has been looked for and not found. If invasion is present, the report must include the measurements of maximum depth of invasion and maximum width of the invasive tumour. It should also stipulate whether lymphatic channels are involved or not, whether the growth pattern is confluent or not, and whether the invasive lesion passes to the edge of the specimen.

3. Whether or not the intraepithelial lesion has been completely excised, at both endocervical or ectocervical extremes. Stripping of epithelium at the edges of the specimen should also be stated, as this would make it impossible to comment on the completeness of excision.

4. A point should be made if no abnormality is found but extensive epithelial loss is present; it is important to distinguish between a negative biopsy and one that is inadequate because of epithelial loss.

5. Other incidental findings, such as papillomavirus infection, congenital transformation zone, squamous metaplasia, microglandular hyperplasia and inflammation should be recorded.

ENDOCERVICAL CURETTAGE

This procedure usually produces multiple tiny fragments of tissue, often with abundant blood and mucus. Fixation should be in Bouin's fluid, and meticulous care must be exercised to ensure that all the material is processed. Step-serial sections are advisable.

TOTAL HYSTERECTOMY

If, perhaps for reasons of coexistent benign gynaecological disease, the patient with cervical intraepithelial neoplasia is treated by hysterectomy rather than more conservatively, the cervix is amputated to produce a piece of tissue approximately 2 cm thick; then, after fixation, this is serially blocked in the same way as a cone biopsy (Fig. 9.6). Also, transverse serial blocking of the adjacent upper segment of the cervix should be carried out.

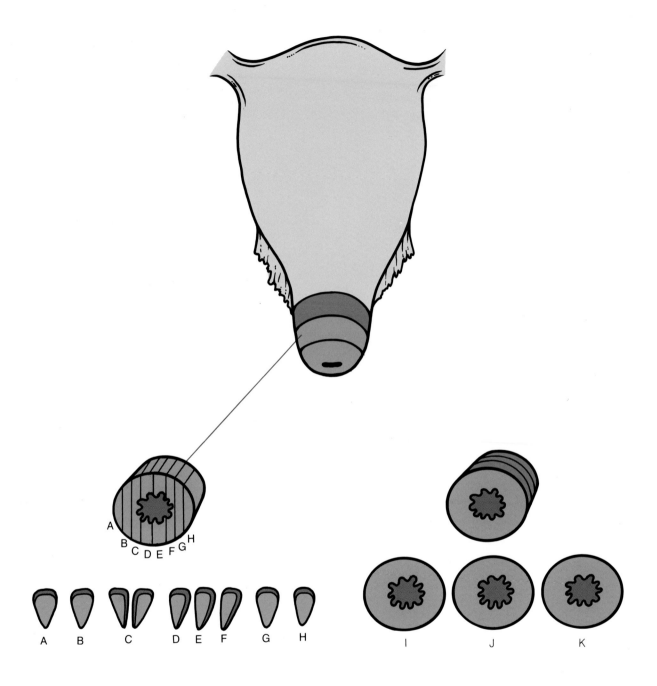

Fig. 9.6 Method of block taking when hysterectomy is performed for cervical intraepithelial neoplasia (or glandular abnormalities). The cervix is amputated in the fresh state, and the adjacent 1.5–2 cm area is removed separately; both specimens are fixed in Bouin's fluid. Serial blocks are taken from the caudal piece in the same way as in a cone biopsy. The cylinder of tissue, through which the canal runs, is serially blocked transversely. The body of the uterus may be blocked in the usual way.

10. Invasive Squamous Disease

STAGING

The complete FIGO staging system for cervical carcinoma is given in Table 10.1. A simplified, diagrammatic representation of the relationships between the subdivisions within stage I is shown in Fig. 10.1. The colposcopist is almost entirely concerned with the preclinical stages of the disease; clinical carcinoma will only be covered in brief.

PRECLINICAL INVASIVE SQUAMOUS CELL CARCINOMA

Preclinical invasive carcinomas may be either stage Ia or stage Ib (see Fig. 10.1). The majority of stage Ib carcinomas are clinically obvious, but preclinical stage Ib invasive carcinoma (formerly referred to as stage Ib [occult]) is an important group to recognize, because of different treatment implications compared with stage Ia carcinoma. Stage Ia invasive squamous cell carcinoma of the cervix is usually referred to as 'microinvasive carcinoma'.

Microinvasive carcinoma

The concept of microinvasive carcinoma was introduced by Mestwerdt in 1947, and it referred to lesions which invaded no more than 5 mm into the cervical stroma, in the belief that these had a better prognosis than the other stage I lesions. Currently, this difference in prognosis and, by implication, treatment of microinvasive carcinomas, as opposed to stage Ib carcinomas, is crucial to our perception of preclinical tumours; can very early invasive carcinoma be treated in a relatively conservative way, and if so, is it possible to define by histology the stage in the growth of the tumour at which radical treatment becomes necessary? This is the question underlying the histological definitions of stage Ia and stage Ib invasive carcinoma of the cervix, which will be discussed after a histological description.

HISTOLOGICAL FEATURES

The earliest stage at which invasion can be recognized is shown in Fig. 10.2. A tiny bud of invasive cells is seen to penetrate the basement membrane and push into the underlying stroma. These cells are similar in morphological appearance to CIN 3 from which they arise.

As invasion becomes more advanced, the cells frequently become better differentiated than the overlying cervical intraepithelial neoplasia (Fig. 10.3).

Table 10.1 1985 modification of FIGO staging of carcinoma of the cervix uteri	
Stage	**Description**
Stage 0	Preinvasive carcinoma (CIN 3, carcinoma in situ).
Stage I	Carcinoma strictly confined to the cervix (extension to the corpus should be disregarded).
Ia	Preclinical carcinomas of the cervix, that is, those diagnosed only by microscopy.
Ia1	Minimal microscopically evident stromal invasion.
Ia2	Lesions detected microscopically that can be measured. The upper limits of the measurement should not show a depth of invasion of more than 5 mm taken from the base of the epithelium, either surface or glandular, from which it originates; and a second dimension, the horizontal spread, must not exceed 7 mm. Larger lesions should be staged as Ib.
Ib	Lesions of greater dimensions than stage Ia2, whether seen clinically or not. Preformed space involvement should not alter the staging but should be recorded specifically to determine whether it should affect treatment decisions in the future.
Stage II	Invasive carcinoma that extends beyond the cervix but has not reached either lateral pelvic wall; involvement of the vagina is limited to the upper two thirds.
Stage III	Invasive carcinoma that extends to either lateral pelvic wall and/or the lower third of the vagina.
Stage IV	Invasive carcinoma that involves urinary bladder and/or rectum or extends beyond the true pelvis.

Schematic representation of the early stages of squamous carcinoma

Stage 0	Stage Ia			Stage Ib	Stages II–IV
CIN 3	Microinvasive carcinoma				Clinical carcinoma
	Stage Ia1 Early stromal invasion	Stage Ia2 Measurable lesions		Stage Ib (formerly occult)	
	Preclinical invasive carcinoma				

Fig. 10.1 Staging of squamous cell carcinoma of the cervix. Schematic representation.

Fig. 10.2 Early stromal invasion. This is the earliest stage of invasion that can be recognized. A small group of cells have breached the smooth contour of the epithelial/stromal junction and invade into the stroma. H&E, x 128.

Fig. 10.3 Early stromal invasion. This example is showing very early invasion which is barely measurable. However, the disruption of the contour of epithelium is clearly seen, and the invasive cells show better differentiation than the matrix cervical intraepithelial neoplasia. This better differentiation is also shown by the cells maturing upwards, towards the surface of the epithelium. H&E, x 32.

There may be a stromal reaction to the infiltrating tumour, characterized by a localized lymphocytic reaction or loosening of the stroma, or both (Figs 10.4 and 10.5).

As invasion progresses even further, other histological features need to be taken into account. These are tumour dimension, lymphatic channel involvement and pattern of growth (Table 10.2).

TUMOUR DIMENSION

It is generally accepted that as the invasion of a preclinical invasive carcinoma in the cervix advances, the prognosis worsens and the need for radical treatment becomes greater. It has been customary to measure invasion only by its depth, but Burghardt has suggested that the tumour volume gives a more reliable indication of prognosis than measurements in only one or even two dimensions. This volumetric assessment necessitates examination of step-serial

Table 10.2   Histological features taken into account in the assessment of early invasive tumours

Tumour dimensions
(measured in two or three dimensions)

Capillary-like space involvement

Growth pattern
(finger-like, spray or confluent)

sections; when the distance between the sections is known, the third dimension can be calculated, in addition to the two dimensions of depth and width in the section which shows the greatest extent of invasion.

Fig. 10.4 Early stromal invasion. Islands of invasive cells, less than 1 mm from their epithelial origins, are surrounded by a dense infiltrate of lymphocytes. H&E, × 32.

Fig. 10.5 Early stromal invasion. There is striking loosening of the stroma surrounding the invasive islands, with a slight increase in the number of lymphocytes. H&E, × 32.

a.   b.   c.

Fig. 10.6 Microinvasive carcinoma. (a) Diagrammatic representation, showing the tumour measurements that need to be taken. **(b)** Measurement of microinvasive carcinoma: this is a section from a hysterectomy specimen in which a preclinical invasive carcinoma was found. **(c)** The superimposed lines indicate the measurements that should be recorded. × 1.

It has been demonstrated that there is no risk of metastatic spread up to 500 mm^3 of tumour size, provided that no vascular invasion is seen. In most laboratories this form of assessment is considered too time consuming, but it is recommended that a two-dimensional (depth and width) measurement of tumour size is given, rather than a measurement of the depth alone (Fig. 10.6).

LYMPHATIC CHANNEL INVOLVEMENT

This can be identified in some preclinical invasive squamous cell carcinomas (Fig. 10.7). It would seem reasonable to argue that a tumour which has lymphatic channel involvement is more likely to have lymph node metastases than one in which such involvement is not seen, implying a worse prognosis and the need for a more radical treatment.

Unfortunately, information on this point is conflicting and hampered by the diversity of lesions that have been accepted as microinvasive. In one often quoted study, Roche and Norris took step-serial sections from 30 cervices which had been diagnosed as containing microinvasive carcinoma, with invasion of 2–5 mm from the surface epithelium; 57% of the patients had 'capillary-like space' involvement. These women had all been treated by radical hysterectomy with pelvic lymphadenectomy, but no metastatic deposits were found in any lymph nodes.

From this study, the authors concluded that the presence of tumour in lymphatic spaces was of no value in predicting which patients were likely to have secondary involvement of lymph nodes.

Nevertheless, subsequent studies have suggested that the presence of lymphatic channel involvement in early invasive carcinoma of the cervix is, indeed, an indication of increased risk of metastases, and this risk becomes greater as the tumour increases in size. The results of these studies indicate that lymphatic channel involvement does not predict an increased risk of pelvic lymph node involvement if invasion is less than 3 mm, but its presence should be taken into account when planning treatment of patients with invasion of 3–5 mm. However, there are individual cases where invasion may be only as much as 2 mm, but with lymphatic channel involvement and pelvic node metastases.

Sometimes the pathologist finds it difficult to decide whether lymphatic channel involvement is present or not; confusion may be caused by tissue shrinkage around invasive buds, leaving a clear space which can be readily mistaken for a lymphatic channel. Only if the nuclei of endothelial cells can be identified should the diagnosis of lymphatic channel involvement be made.

GROWTH PATTERN

The earliest 'finger-like' pattern of growth is illustrated in Figs 10.2–10.5. As the tumour becomes more advanced, this often changes to produce a confluent growth pattern (Fig. 10.8). It has been suggested that the latter is more likely to be associated with metastatic spread, but as this pattern is likely to be seen in more advanced tumours, it may simply be a factor of depth of invasion. Occasionally, multiple

Fig. 10.7 Lymphatic channel involvement. A clump of tumour cells is present within a preformed space. The nuclei of the endothelial cells are easily recognized. H&E, x 128.

Fig. 10.8 Preclinical invasive carcinoma with a confluent growth pattern. This is the same case as in Fig. 10.7. The tumour is invading as a confluent mass of irregular islands, in contrast to the pattern shown in Figs 10.3–10.5. H&E, x 12.8.

finger-like processes of invasion are seen over a wide area, creating a 'spray-like' configuration which is distinct from a confluent pattern (Fig. 10.9).

CYTOLOGICAL FEATURES

The cytological diagnosis of microinvasive carcinoma of the cervix is controversial. Some cytologists believe that a distinction between CIN 3 and the earliest stages of invasive disease cannot be made with cytology. This view is partly supported by the corresponding problems of histological interpretation.

However, there is evidence that, in a significant proportion of cases, it is possible to recognize cytological features which strongly suggest the beginning of invasiveness of a lesion, or at least the point at which the lesion is no longer intraepithelial. The application of cytology in this area is difficult; diligence and experience are required, in order to recognize the subtle changes and interpret them in a meaningful way (Table 10.3).

A striking histological feature of minimal invasion is cytoplasmic differentiation, and this can be recognized with cytology. The cell borders are less well defined than in severe dyskaryosis. The cytoplasm appears more finely granular, frequently staining a pinkish hue (Fig. 10.10), although blue or green staining cytoplasm is also seen. The cytoplasmic differentiation must be distinguished from that associated with human papillomavirus infection; the absence of keratinization and dyskaryosis will allow this distinction on most occasions.

Occasionally the cells assume an elongated or elliptical shape. Odd-shaped cells with tails and rounded projections are sometimes observed. Unlike

Table 10.3 Cytological features associated with microinvasive carcinoma
1 Tendency to form large sheets of cells rather than strings
2 Smaller, paler staining nuclei/cells
3 Cytoplasmic differentiation
4 Small tails and rounded projections to cytoplasm / sometimes keratinised
5 Increased pleomorphism
6 More obvious nuclear 'clearing'
7 Loss of round appearances to cells

cervical intraepithelial neoplasia, where the cells tend to be seen in lines or small groups, in microinvasion the cells tend to appear loosely associated in sheets (Fig. 10.11). The nuclei may show marked pleomorphism and hyperchromasia (Fig. 10.12), but the chromatin may appear less coarsely clumped than in intraepithelial neoplasia, frequently with more obvious nuclear clearing. Variation in intensity of staining between one nucleus and another may also be seen.

As colposcopic recognition of minimal invasive disease is also difficult, it is important that the cytology is carefully reviewed; where cellular features suggest that the lesion is no longer typical of cervical intraepithelial neoplasia, the colposcopist should be alerted to the possibility of invasion by the appropriate wording of the report.

However, it is equally important not to over-diagnose early invasive disease cytologically, as this

Fig. 10.9 Preclinical invasive carcinoma with a confluent growth pattern. Although in this example the maximum depth of invasion is under 2 mm, it is taking place over a broad field and with a confluent, 'spray-like' growth pattern. H&E, x 12.8.

Fig. 10.10 Microinvasive carcinoma. Loosely associated sheets of cells, showing cytoplasmic differentiation staining a pinkish hue. Papanicolaou stain, x 128.

would lead to difficulties in managing the patients, and would also undermine the confidence of clinicians and colposcopists in the cytological opinion.

It is not possible to make a confident distinction between stage Ia and stage Ib invasive carcinoma with cytology.

DEFINITIONS

The search for a definition of microinvasive carcinoma is the quest for the histological features that allow a reliable identification of the maximum disease which can be safely treated in a conservative manner; this ideal definition is not yet available. A Study Group on Preclinical Carcinoma of the Cervix was held at the Royal College of Obstetricians and Gynaecologists in 1981, and the following proposals were made:

Carcinoma of the cervix stage Ia (microinvasive carcinoma) is a histological diagnosis which should be made on a large biopsy removing the whole lesion, preferably a cone biopsy. Two groups should be recog-nized:

(a) **Early stromal invasion** in which invasive buds are present either in continuity with an in situ lesion, or apparently separated cells not more than 1 mm from the nearest surface or crypt basement membrane.

(b) **Measurable lesions** should be measured in two dimensions. The depth should be measured from the base of the epithelium from which it develops, and should not exceed 5 mm. The largest dimension should not exceed 10 mm on the section that shows the greatest extent. When reporting stage Ia lesions, the chosen depth and diameter should be given for inclusion with cases in the statistics. Furthermore, the percentage of confluent lesions and cases with involvement of endothelium-lined spaces (vessels) should be stated.

The International Federation for Gynaecology and Obstetrics has used these recommendations in its most recent changes concerning the staging of cervical carcinoma (see Table 10.1). However, it should be noted that there is a disagreement over the lateral dimension of a lesion to be classified as stage Ia: FIGO requires a maximum of 7 mm, whereas the RCOG Group accepts 10 mm.

Nevertheless, it must be realized that these are only provisional and interim working definitions which, if used by pathologists consistently for several years over a sufficient number of cases, should enable an accurate comparison of treatment results, so as to form the basis of future management. These provisional definitions should, therefore, not be taken as a guide to treatment, but the guidelines should be used in the hope that a more precise definition will eventually emerge which can be directly correlated to management.

Stage Ia lesions are further subdivided into stage Ia1 and stage Ia2. Examples of stage Ia1 lesions are illustrated in Figs 10.2–10.5. These tumours, with invasion of less than 1 mm, have no metastatic potential, and radical treatment is not indicated. The dilemma is over more advanced cases falling into stage Ia2.

Stage Ib lesions are of greater dimensions than stage Ia2, irrespective of whether they are clinically apparent or not.

Fig. 10.11 Microinvasive carcinoma. Loosely associated sheets of cells, with marked pleomorphism and some cytoplasmic tails. Papanicolaou stain, x 128.

Fig. 10.12 Microinvasive carcinoma. Cells are showing hyperchromatic nuclei with clearing. The cytoplasm in some cells has rounded projections. Papanicolaou stain, x 128.

INVASIVE SQUAMOUS CELL CARCINOMA

Gross features

With colposcopy, an early invasive carcinoma of the cervix may appear striking. However, to the unaided eye diagnosis is not always easy to make, as the features are not characteristic. The surface may be slightly raised, and the tumour may present as a rough, red, granular area, bleeding to the touch. There is often little to distinguish an early invasive carcinoma from an ectopy, where vascular endocervical tissue is present on the vaginal part of the cervix.

Many invasive squamous cell carcinomas, by the time they become clinically apparent, are visible on speculum examination and involve the external os. However, some remain entirely within the canal, and although of squamous origin they are clinically classified as endocervical carcinomas. The growth pattern may be either predominantly exophytic, with polypoid or papillary excrescences, or ulcerating with necrosis. Frequently, a combination of these two patterns is seen.

Cytological features

Squamous cell carcinomas are conventionally subdivided into large cell keratinizing carcinoma, large cell non-keratinizing carcinoma, and small cell non-keratinizing carcinoma (Table 10.4). Although, in general terms, the small cell carcinomas are poorly differentiated and the keratinizing carcinomas are well differentiated, the classification given in Table 10.4 describes the cell type rather than the grade; the nuclear grade should also be assessed in this cell

Table 10.4 Classification of squamous cell carcinomas of the cervix

Cell type
Large-cell, keratinizing

Large-cell, non-keratinizing

Small-cell, non-keratinizing

Grade
Grade 1 – well differentiated

Grade 2 – moderately differentiated

Grade 3 – poorly differentiated

type. Some keratinizing carcinomas (Fig. 10.13) may show areas of high nuclear grade.

LARGE CELL KERATINIZING CARCINOMA

This consists of typical epidermoid cells, with characteristic central whorls of cells containing central nests of keratin ('keratin pearls'). Intercellular bridges are seen, along with keratohyaline granules and cytoplasmic keratinization (see Fig. 10.13).

LARGE CELL NON-KERATINIZING CARCINOMA

This is composed of cells which are usually recognizable as being squamous because of their polygonal shape. There may be a little individual cell keratinization, but keratin pearls are absent (Fig. 10.14). These tumours are often, but not necessarily, of a worse nuclear grade than the keratinizing tumours.

Fig. 10.13 Invasive squamous cell carcinoma; large cell keratinizing type. The characteristic keratin pearls are prominent. H&E, x 32.

Fig. 10.14 Invasive squamous cell carcinoma; large cell non-keratinizing type. A moderate lymphocytic infiltrate is present in the stroma. H&E, x 32.

SMALL CELL NON-KERATINIZING CARCINOMA

This consists of small, round cells with fairly uniform, dark nuclei. There is often little to characterize these tumours as squamous, although on rare occasions keratinizing examples are seen (Fig. 10.15). Some tumours, classified as small cell non-keratinizing squamous cell carcinomas, contain argyrophil cells with a pattern resembling the small cell anaplastic ('oat cell') carcinoma of the bronchus (Fig. 10.16). These tumours are associated with a particularly poor prognosis.

Cytological features

The cytological appearances associated with invasive squamous carcinoma have been well described (Table 10.5). However, the reliability of cervical smears in

Table 10.5 Cytological features associated with invasive squamous carcinoma
1 Nuclear pleomorphism
2 Marked anisocytosis and anisonucleosis
3 Occasionally bizarre 'tadpole' and 'spindle' forms
4 Highly keratinized cytoplasm (in some cases)
5 Much associated cell necrosis and debris frequently with red blood cells.

the identification of squamous cell carcinoma of the cervix has been questioned. To some extent this may be related to the experience of the individual cyto-

Fig. 10.15 Invasive squamous cell carcinoma; small cell keratinizing type. (a) This is an unusual variant of squamous cell carcinoma, and is the same example as shown in Figs 10.6b and 10.10. Keratin pearls are

prominent. H&E, x 32. **(b)** The cells appear as a loosely associated group in a blood stained background. Although the nuclei are small, they are notably pleomorphic. Papanicolaou stain, x 128.

Fig. 10.16 Invasive carcinoma; small cell anaplastic type. (a) There are no features to suggest a squamous origin of this tumour, the appearances of which are similar to the small cell anaplastic 'oat cell' carcinoma of the bronchus.

H&E, x 32. **(b)** The nuclei show hyperchromasia and pleomorphism with a homogeneous appearance of chromatin; there is obvious moulding. Papanicolaou stain, x 128.

logist, and also to the mistaken expectation that all invasive disease will present with a large number of bizarre and keratinized malignant cells.

It is certainly true that, in the case of large cell keratinizing carcinoma, the malignant cells are sometimes grossly enlarged, with obvious pleomorphism, and associated with bizarre tadpole or spindle forms which may show excessive keratinization (Fig. 10.17). In the large cell non-keratinizing type, either no evidence of keratinization is seen, or only occasional small keratinized cells are present (Figs 10.18 – 10.20).

However, in a case of squamous cell carcinoma, the cervical smear will quite frequently contain very few malignant cells. Consequently, smears must be carefully screened to pick out the few malignant cells amongst the red blood cells and necrotic debris (Fig. 10.21).

At the other end of the spectrum, cells from a well differentiated lesion may not show bizarre and

Fig. 10.17 Invasive squamous cell carcinoma; large cell keratinizing type. A bizarre, keratinized, multinucleated cell is present in the centre, surrounded by necrotic debris. Papanicolaou stain, x 128.

Fig. 10.18 Invasive squamous cell carcinoma; large cell non-keratinizing type. An irregular sheet of pleomorphic cells with hyperchromatic nuclei and sparse cytoplasm is seen, characteristic of this type of tumour. Papanicolaou stain, x 128.

Fig. 10.19 Invasive squamous cell carcinoma; large cell non-keratinizing type. This group of grossly pleomorphic cells demonstrate a greatly increased nuclear/cytoplasmic ratio. Papanicolaou stain, x 128.

Fig. 10.20 Invasive carcinoma. One elongated, keratinizing 'spindle' form is present, together with discrete, pale staining but pleomorphic cells. Papanicolaou stain, x 128.

keratinized forms but only minimal nuclear change with abundant cytoplasm, and these may closely resemble cells of squamous metaplasia (Fig. 10.22). Cells arising from a small cell anaplastic carcinoma (oat cell type) show moulding of the nuclei (see Fig. 10.16b; Fig. 10.23), very similar to the characteristic appearances of oat cell carcinoma in sputum.

The absence of striking cytoplasmic change may add to the difficulty of recognition. The ability to discriminate between necrotic change associated with

inflammation and that associated with invasive cancer is only improved by careful evaluation both of individual cell changes and overall smear pattern.

Differentiation from human papillomavirus infection depends on identifying the other features seen with that infection. The background and other cell types seen, as well as the distribution of keratinized cells together with dyskeratosis and dyskaryosis, all need to be considered in arriving at a final diagnosis.

Fig. 10.21 Invasive carcinoma. (a) Discrete, poorly displayed malignant cells are seen in a sea of blood stained debris and polymorphonuclear leucocytes. **(b)** One large, pale, necrotic cell in a sea of blood. The nucleus is poorly displayed but is greatly enlarged, with an irregular shape and chromatin pattern. Papanicolaou stain, x 128.

Fig. 10.22 Invasive carcinoma. This small group of cells has well defined, blue-green cytoplasm and enlarged nuclei which do not show bizarre changes. Careful evaluation is required to recognize the more subtle features suggestive of invasion. Papanicolaou stain, x 128.

Fig. 10.23 Small cell anaplastic carcinoma. The two groups of small, densely stained cells show clear evidence of moulding reminiscent of bronchial 'oat cell' carcinoma. Papanicolaou stain, x 128.

COLPOSCOPIC FEATURES

Invasive carcinoma is generally thought of as an area of ulceration or gross and irregular hypertrophy. However, in many instances, the disease will be clinically unsuspected and recognized for the first time when the patient is referred for colposcopy following an abnormal cervical smear.

Colposcopically, atypical vessels are often thought to be the hallmark of an invasive carcinoma. These are focal colposcopic appearances in which the blood vessel pattern shows not as punctation, mosaic or delicately branching vessels, but as irregular vessels with abruptly changing courses, with 'comma', 'corkscrew' or 'spaghetti-like' forms. Atypical vessels are coarser than normal vessels, and are irregular in width, shape and course. They have a horizontal component, and may appear and disappear abruptly.

Even where the cervix is macroscopically normal, wide intercapillary distance, the presence of atypical vessels and an irregular surface, often with ulceration, will alert the colposcopist to the possibility of invasive disease (Figs 10.24–10.30). Nevertheless, many early invasive lesions have no atypical vessels. In a series of 180 patients with preclinical invasive disease (stage Ia and Ib), Beredet and colleagues reported that no markedly atypical vessels were found at colposcopy. The main features associated with invasion were large lesions with complex patterns (i.e. combination of acetowhite, mosaic and punctation), a raised, irregular surface and CIN 3 with cervical canal extensions.

If the lesion is ulcerated, surface epithelium is lost

Fig. 10.24 Microinvasive carcinoma (a) before and (b) after application of acetic acid. The possibility of microinvasion was raised by the irregular, friable epithelium at the '6 o'clock' position. Such lesions require an excisional cone biopsy.

Fig. 10.25 Microinvasive carcinoma (a) before and (b) after application of acetic acid. The lesion demonstrates atypical vessels and a surface which is irregular and friable.

Fig. 10.26 Microinvasive carcinoma and CIN 3. Using the saline technique and a green filter, the vessels are clearly seen. The anterior part of the lesion is showing the coarse punctation pattern of CIN 3. The part of the lesion around the external os displays atypical vessels and an irregular surface. The lesion extends into the canal, and requires an excisional cone biopsy.

Fig. 10.27 Microinvasive carcinoma. Atypical vessels are seen after application of acetic acid.

Fig. 10.28 (a) Microinvasive carcinoma. This was suspected because of the very prominent, coarse punctation, atypical vessels and a surface which is raised

above the adjacent normal squamous epithelium. **(b)** Histology of the same lesion.

Fig. 10.29 Invasive carcinoma. Even without application of acetic acid, the lesion is raised, irregular, friable and contains atypical vessels.

Fig. 10.30 Invasive carcinoma after application of acetic acid.

and there may be a few or even no vessels to be seen in the ulcer cavity. On the other hand, if the lesion is hypertrophic, there is proliferation of epithelial tissue, and the vessels in this instance are usually very prominent. Even in the presence of obvious invasive disease, the cervix and upper vagina should be examined by colposcopy to assess the limits of abnormality. Frequently, unsuspected premalignant disease is found to extend beyond the borders of invasion; it is therefore important that any treatment regimen takes the extent of both malignant and premalignant disease into consideration.

11. Glandular Lesions

HISTOPATHOLOGICAL CLASSIFICATION

Malignant and premalignant changes of the glandular epithelium of the cervix make up a small but important group of diseases. The proportion of patients with adenocarcinoma, reported in various series of cervical carcinoma, ranges between 4.5 and 34%.

More recently, there has been an apparent increase in the proportion of adenocarcinomas. This may be due to a reduction in the number of squamous cell carcinomas, perhaps as a result of screening and treatment at the preinvasive stage, rather than an increase of adenocarcinomas. However, there is some evidence of an absolute increase of cases of adenocarcinoma.

Table 11.1 Classification of adenocarcinoma of the cervix

Cervical cell adenocarcinoma
Mucinous adenocarcinoma
Endometrioid adenocarcinoma
Clear cell carcinoma
Minimal deviation adenocarcinoma
Serous papillary carcinoma
Adenosquamous (mixed) carcinoma
   Mucoepidermoid carcinoma
   Glassy cell carcinoma

Some three decades ago, the observed proportion of adenocarcinomas within the total number of cervical carcinomas encountered was typically in the region of 4–5%. By comparison, in one recent large study using routine data from a British regional cancer registry, adenocarcinomas represented approximately one in six of all cervical invasive malignancies reported, which is a clear and worrying increase. Moreover, almost 8% of those lesions occurred in single women, compared with just over 4% for squamous lesions in the same group.

In another large study of the incidence of adenocarcinoma, using recent data from three British cancer registries and covering a span of 15 years, the number of cases per million in women between 20 and 34 years of age almost tripled (2.4 to 6.6 cases per million): an alarming increase in this young and potentially fertile group. Little change was observed in women aged 35 years and over.

Glandular abnormalities of the cervix may be invasive or intraepithelial; a classification of invasive adenocarcinoma is given in Table 11.1. As the

Fig. 11.1 Adenocarcinoma in situ. (a) At low magnification, the architectural pattern of the endocervical crypts is seen to be undisturbed. H&E, x 12.8. **(b)** The highly abnormal epithelium follows exactly the same contours as the normal epithelium, sharing the same basement membrane. H&E, x 32.

Fig. 11.2 Adenocarcinoma in situ. The contrast between normal and abnormal epithelium is clearly demonstrated. The area of adenocarcinoma in situ demonstrates all the features listed in Table 11.1. H&E, x 128.

Fig. 11.3 Adenocarcinoma in situ.. There are numerous mitotic figures. H&E, x 128.

Table 11.2 Classification of glandular intraepithelial abnormalities of the cervix

Mild glandular atypia   = GIN grade 1

Severe glandular atypia = GIN grade 2

Adenocarcinoma in situ = GIN grade 3

GIN = Glandular intraepithelial neoplasia

Table 11.3 Histological features of glandular intraepithelial neoplasia of the cervix

Architectural features
Often retains normal architectural pattern
Slight crowding is accepted
Slight variation in size and shape of glands is accepted

(If architectural changes are marked, even in the absence of striking cellular changes, or if atypical crypts are found outside the normal crypt field, a diagnosis of invasive carcinoma must be considered)

Cellular changes
Increased nuclear/cytoplasmic ratio
Variation in nuclear size and shape
Mitotic activity
Loss of polarity
Stratification
Reduced mucin production

colposcopist is mainly concerned with preclinical disease, invasive intraepithelial adenocarcinoma will be covered in brief.

Similar to intraepithelial squamous neoplasia, glandular intraepithelial neoplasia appears to form a spectrum of disease, ranging from very mild to severe forms. Various classifications have been suggested; the two most widely used are shown in Table 11.2. The most severe abnormalities are classified as adenocarcinoma in situ, and lesser degrees of change are referred to as glandular atypia, either mild or severe, according to the degree of abnormality.

Alternatively, in an attempt to correlate this classification with that of cervical intraepithelial neoplasia, terms such as glandular intraepithelial neoplasia (GIN) grades 1,2 and 3, have been proposed.

ADENOCARCINOMA IN SITU

Adenocarcinoma in situ (AIS) of the cervix has been recognized for over 30 years. However, it has been reported most frequently in recent years, often in association with squamous cervical intraepithelial neoplasia, or adjacent to an invasive adenocarcinoma.

Microscopically (Table 11.3), adenocarcinoma in situ maintains the architectural pattern of normal endocervical crypts, and often involves only the superficial crypts (Fig. 11.1). The abnormal epithelium shows loss of polarity, increased nuclear size, nuclear pleomorphism and anisokaryosis, mitotic activity, reduction in cytoplasmic mucin and, frequently, stratification (Figs 11.2 and 11.3).

The glandular atypias show the same changes as adenocarcinoma in situ, but to a less marked degree (Figs 11.4 and 11.5). For example, a severe glandular atypia will show fewer mitotic figures, more preservation of polarity, less stratification and more mucin production than an adenocarcinoma in situ (compare

Fig. 11.4 Glandular atypia. Mitotic figures are seen, and there is an increase in nuclear size with some nuclear pleomorphism. However, polarity is largely maintained, and mucin-containing cytoplasm is apparent. H&E, x128.

Fig. 11.5 Glandular atypia. This example shows rather less abnormality than Fig. 11.4. H&E, x 128.

113

Figs 11.2 and 11.4). However, as in cervical intra-epithelial neoplasia, a distinction between the grades of glandular intraepithelial neoplasia is artificial and arbitrary.

Strictly speaking, the term 'adenocarcinoma in situ' should be used only when the crypt architecture is not appreciably altered (see Fig. 11.1).

Even so, some authors show examples of adeno-carcinoma in situ in which there is reduplication and budding of the crypts (Fig. 11.6), sometimes with a 'back-to-back' pattern of the glands (Fig. 11.7). It is very difficult to recognize the beginning of invasion in an adenocarcinoma, as it invades by newly formed glands pushing into the stroma (Fig. 11.8) rather than by cells invading individually or in groups, which is the case with squamous cell carcinoma. This difficulty is compounded by the application of the term 'microinvasive adenocarcinoma', the criteria for which are not equivocal; in our present state of knowledge, there seems little value in using this term.

Distribution of glandular intraepithelial neoplasia

In theory, glandular abnormalities may affect any part or all of the endocervical glandular field of the cervix. However, in practice, most examples of adenocarcinoma in situ are found adjacent to the squamocolumnar junction, affecting both the surface epithelium and the superficial gland crypts. Very few examples have been described in which only deep crypts are involved; their rarity may, of course, be

Fig. 11.6 Adenocarcinoma in situ. The architectural pattern is disturbed, with glandular reduplication and formation of 'tunnel clusters'. H&E, x 32.

Fig. 11.7 As the complexity of the reduplicating glandular structures increases, a 'back-to-back', cribriform pattern develops. It is questionable whether this should be regarded as adenocarcinoma in situ or as invasive adenocarcinoma. H&E, x 32.

Fig. 11.8 Adenocarcinoma in situ, with early invasion. Although a management related category of microinvasive cervical adenocarcinoma is not recognized, very early stromal invasion is seen. There is little disturbance of the architectural pattern, but a stromal response, with some clearing and an increase in lymphocytes, can be seen. This example illustrates that a well differentiated adenocarcinoma invades by producing well formed, new glandular structures. H&E, x 12.8.

due to the fact that they cannot be recognized until a clinical carcinoma develops. Skip lesions are only rarely found.

Glandular and squamous intraepithelial abnormalities: association

As many as 50% of reported cases of adenocarcinoma in situ have been associated with coexistent squamous cervical intraepithelial neoplasia, which raises interesting questions regarding the aetiology and histogenesis of both conditions. However, practical considerations are also posed by this association. Most importantly, a woman may harbour cervical intraepithelial neoplasia together with adenocarcinoma in situ, but there is a chance that only the squamous abnormality will be recognized by cytology and colposcopy.

Failure to diagnose a glandular abnormality may possibly affect the eventual outcome, if conservative treatment is designed solely for the intraepithelial neoplasia. With an increase in the cases of adenocarcinoma in situ being diagnosed, this is a strong argument for using excisional rather than destructive procedures in treating cervical intraepithelial neoplasia.

In situ and invasive adenocarcinomas: relationship

The way in which adenocarcinoma in situ is regarded depends upon whether it is genuinely a premalignant state. Cases of progression of an adenocarcinoma from in situ to invasive have been described. The shortest progression time documented lies in the region of three to seven years, but a period as long as 14 years has been reported. Another less strongly supportive observation is that the average age at diagnosis is around 15–18 years less than the average for adenocarcinoma.

There is one small study of women with adenocarcinoma where antecedent cervical cytology smears were available for further scrutiny. In six out of 13 cases, atypical glandular cells were evidently being exfoliated over an interval of two to eight years before the adenocarcinoma became obvious. It seems unlikely that a covert adenocarcinoma would have remained asymptomatic for so long, which implies that it was preceded by a non-invasive precursor yielding the atypical cells. Strong evidence supporting a progression from in situ to invasive adenocarcinoma is the finding of the former at the periphery of an invasive adenocarcinoma, and also the earlier stage of a field of predominantly in situ adenocarcinoma with unjustifiable invasion.

Finally, in support of adenocarcinoma in situ and cervical glandular atypia being the precursors of

Fig. 11.9 HMFG1 expression. (a) Normal cervical columnar epithelium (cuticular expression only).
(b) Cervical glandular atypia (cuticular and cytoplasmic expression) on the right, with H&E section for morphology on the left. Immunoperoxidase staining; reaction product is brown. Courtesy of Dr Michael Wells, Leeds.

adenocarcinoma, there are some recent studies of human milk fat globulin (HMFG1; Fig. 11.9), c-*myc* oncogene expression and amplification (Fig. 11.10), and silver staining nucleolar organizer regions (AgNORs; Fig. 11.11) in the cancer and putative precursors. The presence and pattern of expression were similar, suggesting a relationship.

Fig. 11.10 c-*myc* oncogene amplification. Normal columnar epithelium (above left), and adenocarcinoma in situ (below right). Immunoperoxidase staining; reaction product is brown.

INVASIVE ADENOCARCINOMA

Various histological patterns may be seen in invasive adenocarcinoma of the cervix (see Table 11.1). These patterns are not mutually exclusive, and some tumours may have diverse histological appearances in different parts of the cervix.

Endocervical tumour

This is the most common type of cervical tumour, accounting for up to 90% in some series. The glands are of variable sizes and shapes, showing budding and branching. The epithelium generally resembles normal endocervical epithelium (Fig. 11.12).

Adenoma malignum

The terms 'adenoma malignum' and 'minimal deviation adenocarcinoma' have been used to describe a carcinoma in which the architectural pattern is particularly well differentiated. Moreover, there is virtually no atypia of the epithelial cells, which show normal polarity and very little mitotic activity (Fig. 11.13). Histological features do not reflect the biologi-

Fig. 11.11 Silver staining nucleolar organizer regions (AgNORs) in nuclei. (a) Normal columnar epithelium (low dot counts); **(b)** adenocarcinoma in situ (high dot counts); **(c)** invasive adenocarcinoma (high dot counts). Silver staining technique; reaction product is black.

cal behaviour of these tumours, and prognosis is poor.

Mucinous and papillary tumours

These tumours have the appearances that their names imply. The mucinous tumour is composed of cells of enteric type, with abundant mucin-rich cytoplasm and basal nuclei. The papillary pattern is rarely seen as a pure variant, and is usually associated with other patterns; it is composed of complex papillary fronds, supported by fibrovascular cores.

Clear cell carcinoma

This carcinoma is morphologically the same as the more common clear cell tumours of the ovary and endometrium, and has been extensively studied because of its development in the daughters of women who were given diethylstilboestrol in pregnancy. It comprises a variety of different patterns: solid, clear cell, tubulocystic and papillary areas, and 'hobnail' epithelium (Figs 11.14 and 11.15). Only about 2% of cervical carcinomas belong to this category.

Endometrioid carcinoma

This has the same appearances as the common type of endometrial carcinoma. Diagnosis can only be made if the endometrium itself is normal, and is best made on a complete hysterectomy specimen. Also, the distinction is possible only on a fairly well differentiated tumour.

Fig. 11.12 Invasive adenocarcinoma of the cervix: cervical cell type. H&E, x 32.

Fig. 11.13 Invasive adenocarcinoma of cervix: minimal deviation type. There is some irregularity of the glandular architecture of the tumour which is deeply invasive. However, the epithelium is indistinguishable from normal epithelium. H&E, x 32.

Fig. 11.14 Invasive adenocarcinoma of the cervix: clear cell type. A tubulocystic area is seen, in which 'hobnail' cells are prominent. H&E, x 32.

Fig. 11.15 Invasive adenocarcinoma of the cervix: clear cell type. A papillary area is seen. H&E, x 32.

CYTOLOGY OF GLANDULAR LESIONS OF THE CERVIX

The cytological assessment of glandular lesions is hampered by a lack of knowledge regarding the significance and natural history of intraepithelial abnormalities, and uncertainty over the earliest stages of invasive disease (see above). The absence of precise histological guidelines in some of these areas also adds to the difficulty of a cytological interpretation.

Adenocarcinoma of the cervix

This is not often recognized by cytologists. The recognition of individual cell changes is difficult. An experienced cytologist will be able to recognize them when the features are pronounced and noticeably at variance with the normal. Furthermore, if changes occur only in the crypts deep to the surface epithelium, the abnormal cells are unlikely to appear in a cervical smear in significant numbers, if at all. When the surface epithelium is involved, the possibility of obtaining the abnormal glandular cells is, of course, improved.

CYTOLOGICAL FEATURES

The cytological features of adenocarcinoma are nuclear pleomorphism, often with hyperchromasia, irregular chromatin distribution, and occasionally prominent nucleoli (Figs 11.16 and 11.17). Sometimes the nuclei may appear very uniform in size and shape, but one single nucleus may be several times the size of the others (Fig. 11.18).

In a minority of cases, the cells appear as discrete, tightly packed groups with small, densely stained nuclei (Fig. 11.19). The malignant glandular cells

Fig. 11.16 Adenocarcinoma. Cells are showing marked pleomorphism, with obvious nuclear hyperchromasia. The cytoplasm is indistinct and stains blue. Papanicolaou stain, x 128.

Fig. 11.17 Adenocarcinoma. A small cluster of cells is seen, with obvious pleomorphism and occasional prominent nucleoli. One or two cells retain a distinct columnar shape. Papanicolaou stain, x 128.

Fig. 11.18 Adenocarcinoma. A tightly packed sheet of cells, with nuclei of much the same shape and intensity of staining, but one or two nuclei in the centre show marked enlargement. The chromatin pattern is grossly abnormal. Papanicolaou stain, x 128.

Fig. 11.19 Adenocarcinoma. In this example, a few well defined groups of malignant cells are seen. Nuclei are small and darkly stained, without obvious pleomorphism, but with pseudostratification. Papanicolaou stain, x 128.

most frequently appear in sheets and small groups, sometimes in very large numbers (Fig. 11.20). Occasionally, only discrete single cells or small clusters are seen, known as the 'rosette' formation. Pseudostratification of cells within a group is a common appearance.

The cytoplasm is usually poorly defined, finely vacuolated and granular, and cell borders are indistinct (Fig. 11.21). The cells may have an appreciable amount of cytoplasm or virtually none. Not infrequently, endocervical cells showing the whole spectrum of changes can be observed in a single smear: from cells of normal appearance, through those showing nuclear changes not sufficiently marked to suggest malignancy, to cells showing unequivocal malignant features.

Since a histological distinction between adenocarcinoma in situ and invasive adenocarcinoma is made on the architectural features alone, cyto-logically it is virtually impossible to differentiate between the two. Although some authors claim that certain cytological features can be used to distinguish reliably between in situ and invasive adenocarcinoma, a diagnosis from the appearances in a cervical smear should initially be regarded as suggesting an invasive lesion, and an appropriate diagnostic procedure, usually a cone biopsy, should be undertaken.

On rare occasions, the cytological features may be sufficiently obvious to suggest that the malignant cells arise from a mucinous, papillary or endometrioid subtype. However, it is generally not possible to make such distinctions, except perhaps in the case of the clear cell variant which can be cytologically recognized and differentiated. This is characterized by a clear zone in the cytoplasm surrounding the nucleus (Fig. 11.22), and by the nucleus containing a prominent nucleolus (Fig. 11.23).

Fig. 11.20 Adenocarcinoma. In this example, large, dense papillary fragments of malignant and benign glandular cells are seen. Papanicolaou stain, x 32.

Fig. 11.21 Adenocarcinoma. Small cells with nuclear hyperchromasia and irregular chromatin distribution. The cytoplasm is poorly defined and granular, with indistinct cell borders. Papanicolaou stain, x 128.

Fig. 11.22 Adenocarcinoma. In the clear cell variant, the cells characteristically appear in small clusters with prominent nucleoli. Papanicolaou stain, x 128.

Fig. 11.23 Adenocarcinoma. The clear perinuclear zone, characteristic of clear cell carcinoma, is well shown in this small cluster of cells. Papanicolaou stain, x 128.

Lesser degrees of glandular abnormality

It is very difficult to recognize cytologically the lesser degrees of glandular abnormality, i.e. the glandular atypias. These need to be distinguished from adeno-carcinoma in situ, as well as from variants of the normal state. The cytological features of this group are generally the same as those described above for adenocarcinoma, but changes are much less marked.

With cytology, it is often possible to recognize and differentiate the minor degrees of glandular intra-epithelial neoplasia; for instance, those associated with intrauterine contraceptive devices (Fig. 11.24) or inflammation (Fig. 11.25), where the cytoplasm may show eosinophilia and the nuclei are enlarged with some anisonucleosis but minimal chromatin disturbance. Apart from these cases, the role of cytology has yet to be ascertained, as it is in this area that least is known of the significance of abnormalities. A careful study of these minor lesions is needed, to establish criteria which can be applied with sufficient confidence in determining management.

The cytology of glandular abnormalities of the cervix remains a poorly defined but challenging area. However, it must be appreciated that, at present, cervical cytology cannot be regarded as a screening method for these changes, although it is fortunate when glandular lesions are detected in the course of screening for squamous abnormalities.

Cytological differential diagnosis

The cytological distinction between severely dyskary-otic squamous cells and cells arising from an adeno-carcinoma can be difficult (Fig. 11.26), and on occasions impossible. The main differences are listed in Table 11.4.

Endometrial adenocarcinoma can also be confused with endocervical adenocarcinoma. However, a distinction is often possible as the cells from an endometrial adenocarcinoma tend to be smaller and more densely stained, with a more coarsely clumped chromatin and less cytoplasm than is seen in an endocervical adenocarcinoma (Fig. 11.27). Reference to the patient's age and clinical data may also prove helpful (Table 11.5).

Histologically, microglandular hyperplasia is a recognized entity, but the distinguishing cytological features remain elusive (see Chapter 17).

Table 11.4 Differential cytological features of cervical adenocarcinoma and CIN3

Cervical adenocarcinoma	Cervical intra-epithelial neoplasia
1 Indistinct cytoplasm	1 Well defined cytoplasm
2 Pale stained nuclei	2 Hyperchromatic nuclei
3 Subtle nuclear changes	3 Gross nuclear changes
4 Small clusters or large sheets	4 Strings of cells

Fig. 11.24 Atypical glandular cells associated with intrauterine contraceptive device. There is nuclear enlargement, with prominent nucleoli and variation in nuclear size. However, the chromatin is regular in distribution and finely granular. Papanicolaou stain, x 128.

Fig. 11.25 Atypical glandular cells. These are showing binucleation and nuclear enlargement, with prominent nucleoli. There is some eosinophilia and thickening of the cytoplasm, probably reflecting inflammatory changes of little significance. Papanicolaou stain, x 128.

Table 11.5 Distinguishing cytological features between adenocarcinoma and cervical adenocarcinoma

Endometrial	Endocervical
1 Small clusters	1 Larger clusters or sheets
2 Little cytoplasm	2 Larger cells
3 Darkly stained, coarse chromatin	3 Less coarsely clumped chromatin
4 Occasional cytoplasmic vacuoles	4 Rarely vacuolated cytoplasm
5 Blood and debris	5 Occasional giant nuclei

Table 11.6 Cervical glandular 'deviations'

Müllerian metaplasias
   Ciliated cell (tubal)
   Endometrial
Inflammatory changes
Adenomatoid proliferation
Microglandular endocervical hyperplasia
Arias–Stella change
Mesonephric remnants

DIFFERENTIAL DIAGNOSIS OF GLANDULAR LESIONS

A number of glandular 'deviations' may be found in the cervix, and these are shown in Table 11.6. It is important that histopathologists, cytologists and colposcopists are aware of these patterns and do not mistake them for malignant change, either intraepithelial or invasive.

Müllerian 'metaplasias'

The epithelium of the female genital tract, which lines the fallopian tubes, endometrium, endocervix and ectocervix, is embryologically derived from the müllerian (paramesonephric) duct.

Although the typical epithelium of each site is characteristic of that site, apparently inappropriate müllerian epithelium may be found in any position within the tract. Thus, although cervical epithelium is predominantly composed of tall, columnar, mucin secreting cells with basal nuclei (typical endocervical epithelium), occasional glands, or groups of glands, lined by epithelium of the ciliated (tubal) or endometrial type may be found.

Similarly, ciliated cells may be seen within the fallopian tubes. These variants of müllerian epithelium should not be considered abnormal, or even strictly metaplastic, as they represent only a slightly inappropriate müllerian differentiation.

Fig. 11.26 Adenocarcinoma and CIN 3. This illustrates the important differences in shape, size and staining quality between squamous (right) and cervical glandular (left) cells. Papanicolaou stain, x 128. See also Table 11.4.

Fig. 11.27 Cervical and endometrial adenocarcinomas. The cell group on the left demonstrates the small, tightly clustered and densely stained endometrial cells associated with endometrial adenocarcinoma. This is in contrast to the larger, less closely associated but obviously glandular shaped cells of endocervical adenocarcinoma (right). Papanicolaou stain, x 128.

121

Examples of ciliated and endometrial epithelium in the endocervix are shown in Figs 11.28–11.31. Both epithelial types run a risk of being misinterpreted as glandular atypia, because of the different arrangement of nuclei within the cells and overall darker appearance of the epithelium, compared with the normal, mucin secreting endocervical epithelium.

Mitotic activity is not seen in the ciliated epithelium, but it may be found in the endometrial type.

Inflammatory changes

In the presence of severe inflammation in the cervix, the glandular epithelium may show some nuclear changes; in particular, slight nuclear enlargement and pleomorphism (Figs 11.32 and 11.33). These changes may pose serious problems in the distinction from genuine atypia. The changes are usually mild, with no reduction of cytoplasm or mitotic activity.

Fig. 11.28 Ciliated cell metaplasia. This usually affects a small group of glands, which appear dark. H&E, x 12.8.

Fig. 11.29 Ciliated cell metaplasia. The benign nature of ciliated cells is apparent at high magnification. The rather haphazard polarity of the nuclei may initially cause confusion with adenocarcinoma in situ. H&E, x 128.

Fig. 11.30 Endometrial 'metaplasia'. H&E, x 12.8.

Fig. 11.31 Endometrial 'metaplasia'. The presence of mitotic figures and haphazard polarity of the cells sometimes makes difficult the distinction from adenocarcinoma in situ. H&E, x 128.

Adenomatoid proliferation

The histological pattern is common (Figs 11.34 and 11.35). The apparent proliferation of glandular elements, combined with dilatation, gives an appearance that may be confused with hyperplasia or even neoplasia. However, the condition is most probably the result of blockage of the outlet of crypts, and is of no significance; the crypts are generally lined by flattened, inactive epithelium.

Microglandular endocervical hyperplasia

This is a common proliferative state of endocervical epithelium, usually associated with pregnancy or progestagen administration. It will be described in detail in Chapter 17.

Arias-Stella change

This is another pregnancy related phenomenon, and will be described in Chapter 18.

Fig. 11.32 Inflammatory change. An irregular gland is surrounded by stroma which is densely infiltrated by polymorphs and plasma cells. H&E, x 32.

Fig. 11.33 Inflammatory change. The nuclei are enlarged but lack detail. Abundant eosinophilic cytoplasm is present. Mitotic figures are not seen. H&E, x 12.8.

Fig. 11.34 Adenomatoid proliferation. Multiple reduplication of dilated glands is the hallmark of this condition. H&E, x 32.

Fig. 11.35 Adenomatoid proliferation. The glands are lined by flattened, inactive epithelium, and contain mucin. H&E, x 32.

Mesonephric remnants

The remnants of the vestigial mesonephric (Wolffian) duct enter the lateral part of the cervix approximately at the level of the internal cervical os. They pass

Fig. 11.36 Mesonephric remnants. At low magnification, these are seen as scattered collections of rounded and slightly irregular tubules. Often, as in this example, the main duct is seen as a larger, slit-like space. H&E, x 12.8.

through the cervical mesenchyme and into the vaginal wall, continuing as Gärtner's ducts. These may be identified deep within the fibromuscular tissue of the cervix, as rather nondescript collections of tubules lined by 'bland' cuboidal cells (Figs 11.36 and 11.37).

On occasion, these mesonephric remnants may become particularly prominent and hyperplastic (Fig. 11.38). It is important that they are recognized as such and not mistaken for malignancy. It is thought that only very rarely do genuine mesonephric carcinomas arise from these structures in the cervix.

COLPOSCOPIC ASSESSMENT

Adenocarcinoma in situ

This lesion has been receiving increasing attention during the 1980s. Adenocarcinoma in situ has no typical colposcopic appearance. However, some colposcopists have noted that the tips of columnar epithelial villi can appear acetowhite, which may be

Fig. 11.37 Mesonephric remnants. The round or oval spaces are lined by benign, cuboidal epithelium. H&E, x 32.

Fig. 11.38 Hyperplasia of mesonephric remnants. Occasionally, these remnants occupy a large area within the cervical fibromuscular stroma. H&E, x 32.

Fig. 11.39 Adenocarcinoma before (a) and after (b) application of acetic acid. The lesion is relatively small. It is markedly raised and shows atypical vessels. Such a lesion demands a cone biopsy, or at the very least, an excisional biopsy. Squamous carcinoma may exhibit the same features.

the first sign, but this is not a constant feature. It has also been observed that adenocarcinoma in situ may have a flat and densely acetowhite surface which is remarkably fragile and strips as soon as it is touched during the examination.

Adenocarcinoma

As with invasive squamous carcinoma, this lesion is characterized by atypical vessels, irregularity of the surface, and areas suggestive of ulceration. However, the colposcopist will sometimes also find areas with enlarged columnar villi adherent to each other, giving an appearance somewhat similar to that seen in a papillomavirus-induced exophytic papilloma. A number of such areas on the cervix will give it a 'cauliflower' appearance, and the papillae or villi will be very marked (Figs 11.39 – 11.41).

Adenosquamous carcinoma

A combined adenosquamous lesion is currently being diagnosed more frequently than it has been in the

Fig. 11.40 Adenocarcinoma. At low power **(a)** this is an obvious carcinoma. At high power **(b)** the lesion is friable and raised, and exhibits atypical vessels.

Fig. 11.41 Adenocarcinoma. (a) The cervical cytology suggests this diagnosis. **(b & c)** The diagnosis was confirmed on biopsy.

past, primarily because of the pathologists' awareness that squamous invasive carcinoma often has an adenocarcinoma component which can be recognized with the use of appropriate stains. The combined lesion has no characteristic colposcopic appearances.

MANAGEMENT OF GLANDULAR ATYPIAS AND ADENOCARCINOMA IN SITU

This topic is addressed in Chapter 13.

12. Inflammatory and Infective Conditions of the Cervix

CYTOLOGICAL INTRODUCTION

The problems surrounding 'inflammation', perhaps more than any other area of cytology, have given rise to considerable controversy and discussion over recent years.

Inflammatory changes in themselves are of little significance. In strictly pathological terms, cells affected by inflammation show cloudy swelling or necrosis, as a result of cell damage. These cellular appearances may be accompanied by increased numbers of polymorphonuclear leucocytes or lymphocytes and macrophages, depending on the duration of the condition, and are the same whatever the cause of the inflammatory response.

Acute inflammation

In smears taken from an acutely inflamed cervix, an inflammatory exudate is seen with debris and sometimes bacteria, together with numerous polymorphonuclear leucocytes. It is important to exclude physiological causes for the increased polymorphonuclear leucocytes; the pre- and postmenstrual phase, cervical ectropion, pregnancy and the oral contraceptive pill will normally produce an increase in the number of polymorphonuclear leucocytes.

Epithelial cells in inflammation may show enlargement and appear 'bloated' due to cloudy swelling (Fig. 12.1) and necrosis, which appears as pyknosis and karyorrhexis (Fig. 12.2).

Often, the staining reaction will be altered and the smear will show excessive eosinophilia. In smears from premenopausal women there may be increased parabasal cells, as a result of sloughing of superficial

Table 12.1 Causes of inflammatory and degenerative changes of the cervix

Bacteria
Viruses
Trauma
Surgery
Chemical agents
Radiotherapy
Vitamin deficiency (e.g. follate depletion)

layers. In postmenopausal women there may also be an increase in intermediate and superficial squamous cells, possibly associated with the increased vascularity.

Nuclear enlargement of the endocervical glandular cells may be seen, with prominent multiple chromocentres and occasionally nucleoli, multinucleation and mitotic figures. The distinction between inflammatory changes and glandular intraepithelial neoplasia is difficult (see Chapter 11, for a more detailed discussion).

Chronic inflammation

Chronic cervicitis is associated with healing and repair; regenerative changes in cells are discussed in Chapter 14. Cytologically, the pattern is mixed, showing the same degenerative changes seen in acute inflammation together with the features of regeneration (Fig. 12.3). Increased numbers of lymphocytes may be seen with polymorphonuclear leucocytes, but the plasma cells that are usually so prominent in the stroma of histological sections are

Fig. 12.1 Acute inflammation. Cells are showing cloudy swelling associated with early inflammatory response. The cells appear bloated, with eosinophilia. Papanicolaou stain, x 128.

Fig. 12.2 Acute inflammation. Some cells are showing cloudy swelling as in Fig. 12.1. There is pyknosis and karyorrhexis, with cytoplasmic eosinophilia. Polymorphonuclear leucocytes are also present. Papanicolaou stain, x 128.

rarely identified in cervical smears.

In the cervix, the inflammatory response is most commonly associated with bacterial infections (often a result of the toxins produced, rather than the organisms themselves), or viral infections. However, other situations may give rise to degenerative and inflammatory changes in the cells, and it is important for cytologists to be aware of them (Table 12.1).

HUMAN PAPILLOMAVIRUS

Introduction

Since the mid 1970s, human papillomavirus infection

Fig. 12.3 Chronic inflammation. Numerous polymorphonuclear leucocytes are seen, with lymphocytes and degenerative inflammatory changes as in Figs 12.1 and 12.2. The cells in the centre are showing regenerative changes, with enlarged, hyperchromatic nuclei. Papanicolaou stain, x 128.

has been proposed as an aetiological agent in cervical neoplasia. This aspect has been fully discussed in Chapter 3, and therefore only the morphological effects of infection with human papillomavirus will be considered here.

The human papillomavirus produces two types of lesion on the cervix: the condyloma acuminatum, and a flat lesion which has been described as a 'flat wart', non-condylomatous cervical papillomavirus infection, or subclinical papillomavirus infection. Colposcopically, the latter is obvious only after application of aqueous acetic acid.

Cytological features

Koilocytotic atypia, a term first used by Koss and Durfee in 1956, is the feature that has been linked most frequently with subclinical papillomavirus infection.

The cytological features associated with human papillomavirus infection are shown in Table 12.2. The koilocyte is generally accepted as being pathognomonic of this infection, but DNA hybridization studies have shown that koilocytes are only identified in 50–70% of these infections.

The koilocyte has an enlarged nucleus which shows an irregular distribution of nuclear chromatin, surrounded by a large, irregularly shaped halo. The margin of the halo shows cytoplasmic condensation and appears more darkly stained, with a well defined edge (Fig. 12.4).

Keratinized cells, both nucleate and anucleate (Fig. 12.5), are most commonly seen in sheets or plaques with poorly defined cell borders (Fig. 12.6). Although closely associated with human papilloma-

Fig. 12.4 Human papillomavirus infection. A group of koilocytes are showing enlarged nuclei, with minimal chromatin disturbance and prominent perinuclear halos of irregular shapes. Papanicolaou stain, x 128.

Fig. 12.5 Human papillomavirus infection. Keratinized and anucleate keratinized squamous cells.

virus infection, these cells may also be seen in any specific and non-specific inflammatory response.

Multinucleation, most usually binucleation, is frequently seen (Fig. 12.7). Dyskeratosis or individual cell keratinization is another feature (Fig. 12.8); the cells are discrete and often small, with highly keratinized cytoplasm and small, dense nuclei, sometimes showing pyknosis and karyorrhexis.

Overall, the smear may be poorly stained with a 'washed out' appearance (Fig. 12.9), possibly due to acantholysis, and extensive degenerative inflammatory changes. The degree of nuclear aberration may be difficult to assess and differentiate from that of dyskaryotic change. In this instance, the smear should be classified as showing borderline nuclear change. Even so, the interpretation of nuclear changes can give rise to difficulties of over- and underdiagnosis, and the recommended policy of referral for colposcopy after two smears showing borderline change should be adhered to.

With careful evaluation and application of criteria, an accurate assessment can be made in most instances; therefore, a distinction between changes associated with human papillomavirus infection and those of cervical intraepithelial neoplasia is possible. It is important to grade a smear in terms of the degree of dyskaryotic change present, and to recommend management accordingly.

Condyloma acuminatum

HISTOLOGY

In the past, condylomata acuminata of the cervix

Fig. 12.6 Human papillomavirus infection. Keratinized squamous cells, showing minimal nuclear changes and poorly defined cell borders. Papanicolaou stain, x 128.

Fig. 12.7 Human papillomavirus infection. A single multinucleated squamous cell is seen, of the type frequently associated with this infection. Note that the nuclei may touch or overlap but without moulding one another, as opposed to herpes simplex virus. Papanicolaou stain, x 128.

Fig. 12.8 Human papillomavirus infection. Discrete, highly keratinized or dyskeratotic cells, with pyknotic and karyorrhexic nuclei. Papanicolaou stain, x 128.

Fig. 12.9 Koilocytes and multinucleated cells, showing an overall 'washed out' appearance. Papanicolaou stain, x 128.

were considered rare. However, in recent years, and particularly with the increasing use of colposcopy, these lesions have been frequently seen but are still not regarded as common.

Characteristically, condylomata are multiple, and examination will reveal further, perhaps very small, lesions on the cervix, vagina or vulva. Histological examination shows papillomatosis, acanthosis, parakeratosis and hyperkeratosis (Fig. 12.10). At a higher magnification (Fig. 12.11), koilocytotic atypia is a usual feature, as is individual cell keratinization (dyskeratosis) and multinucleation. Often there is a chronic inflammatory infiltrate in the underlying cervical stroma.

Condylomata are frequently associated with cervical intraepithelial neoplasia, and therefore histological examination should include an assessment of atypia in the lesion itself, as well as in the surrounding epithelium; it is not uncommon for a condyloma to contain cells with sufficient atypia to warrant a diagnosis of CIN 2.

COLPOSCOPY

Condylomata are exophytic and, depending on their size, they may be obvious to the naked eye. They usually present as soft, pink or white vascular tumours with multiple, fine, finger-like projections on the surface (Fig. 12.12).

Genital human papillomavirus should be viewed as a field change, involving a large area of similarly derived squamous epithelium. As well as the entire length of the female lower genital tract, the epithelium most at risk extends posteriorly to include

Fig. 12.10 Cervical condyloma acuminatum, affecting the transformation zone. The striking acanthosis and papillomatosis are apparent. Each frond bears a central capillary. H&E, x 12.8.

Fig. 12.11 Cervical condyloma acuminatum. Koilocytotic change is present in groups of superficial cells; the basal cells in this example show no atypia. H&E, x 32.

Fig. 12.12 Cervical condylomata acuminata. (a) Before application of acetic acid. Finger-like projections with a

central capillary are seen. **(b)** After application of acetic acid. Pronounced acetowhite change is seen.

131

the perianal, anal and rectal regions (Figs 12.13 and 12.14).

Presentation is not uncommonly multicentric, involving any combination or even all of these sites which must be examined to prevent reinfection from undiagnosed lesions. The vulva is most commonly involved (Fig. 12.15a), and exophytic cervical condyloma acuminatum will be seen in 5–10% of such cases (Fig. 12.15b). Moreover, women with vulval warts are at increased risk of associated cervical intra-epithelial neoplasia: colposcopic differentiation of the effects of human papillomavirus and those of cervical intraepithelial neoplasia at all sites may be difficult (see below). Cervical cytology and colposcopy are, therefore, mandatory in the management of women with warts in the lower genital tract, or indeed in the perianal/rectal region. Because of the sexually trans-missible nature of this infection, cytology and colposcopy should, if possible, also be offered to the female partners of men with penile warts.

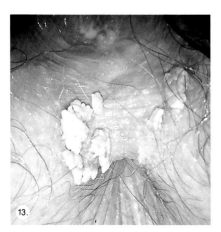

Fig. 12.13 Perianal condylomata acuminata.

Fig. 12.14 (a) Anal intraepithelial neoplasia (AIN 3), showing ulceration. (b) Histology.

Fig. 12.15 (a) Vulval warts. (b) Extended colposcopy, showing a large cervical wart and subclinical papillomavirus infection after application of acetic acid.

Fig. 12.16 Cervical condyloma. Before application of acetic acid: finger-like projections with central capillary loop are seen.

Under the colposcope, cervical condylomata have a typical appearance, with a vascular papilliferous or frond-like surface, each element of which contains a central capillary (Fig. 12.16). After application of acetic acid, there is blanching of the surface and usually definitive acetowhite change, which may persist for some time (see Fig. 12.12). The lesion may be single or multiple, and may be located within or outside the transformation zone (Fig. 12.17).

Occasionally, the surface of the condyloma may have a whorled, heaped up appearance resembling the cerebral cortex, known as 'encephaloid' (Fig. 12.18), or the surface of the lesion may be overtly hyperkeratotic (Fig. 12.19). It should be stressed that a histological diagnosis should be obtained in every case. Sometimes, these lesions may be mimicked by a carcinoma (Fig. 12.20) or, rarely, by a verrucous carcinoma (Fig. 12.21).

Fig. 12.17 Small, solitary cervical condyloma.

Fig. 12.18 Brain-like texture of a cervical condyloma, of the 'encephaloid' type.

Fig. 12.19 Cervical condyloma, with a dense hyperkeratotic surface. No application of acetic acid.

Fig. 12.20 Raised lesion on the posterior lip of the cervix; cervical carcinoma. (a) Before application of acetic acid. **(b)** After application of acetic acid. The typical features of invasion are seen, with a halo of cervical intraepithelial neoplasia and microinvasive disease anteriorly.

Fig. 12.21 Rare verrucous carcinoma in the posterior fornix. This patient had been treated for CIN 3. The lesion could be easily confused with an encephaloid condyloma.

133

Subclinical papillomavirus infection

HISTOLOGY

Subclinical papillomavirus infection presents as flat lesions which cannot usually be detected at naked eye examination. The histological features are listed in Table 12.2, and are illustrated in Figs 12.22–12.24.

The koilocyte is a cell which has a prominent space around the nucleus, with extensive margination of the cytoplasm, giving a sharp edge to the halo. The nuclei of these cells are irregular and hyperchromatic, and those near the surface show wrinkling of the nuclear membrane. The nuclei are usually larger than those of the adjacent, non-ballooned cells (see Fig. 12.23).

Table 12.2 Histological and cytological features of human papillomavirus infection

Koilocytotic change
Multinucleation (usually binucleation)
Dyskeratosis (individual cell keratinization)
Parakeratosis
Acanthosis
Papillomatosis
Appearances possibly due to acantholysis
Keratinized squamous cells
Anucleate keratinized squamous cells

Fig. 12.22 Subclinical papillomavirus infection. Although not a clinical condyloma, this example shows acanthosis with some papillomatosis. Even at this low magnification, koilocytotic change is obvious. H&E, x 32.

Fig. 12.23 Koilocytotic change. A group of cells contain irregular, hyperchromatic, slightly enlarged nuclei which are surrounded by a clear halo. H&E, x 128.

Fig. 12.24 Individual cell keratinization and multinucleation. In addition to koilocytotic change, four cells are showing individual cell keratinization (arrows), and a further cell is binucleate (arrow). H&E, x 128.

Fig. 12.25 Coexistent subclinical papillomavirus infection and cervical intraepithelial neoplasia. Subclinical papillomavirus infection is affecting the surface epithelium on the right, and cervical intraepithelial neoplasia is affecting both the surface epithelium on the left and part of the gland crypt on the lower part of the field. H&E, x 32.

It is important that koilocytotic atypia is not confused with the 'basket weave' pattern of the normal, mature squamous epithelium. The two other main histological features of subclinical papillomavirus infection are individual cell keratinization (dyskeratosis) and multinucleation (usually binucleation; see Fig. 12.24).

Other features which have been described are parakeratosis, frequent mitotic figures, acanthosis, prominent rete pegs and blood vessels surrounded by a little stroma reaching up to the surface.

The histological features of subclinical papillomavirus infection and cervical intraepithelial neoplasia may be combined in two ways (Figs 12.25–12.27): first, both conditions may occur separately in adjacent areas of the epithelium, a pattern frequently seen colposcopically (see Fig. 12.25). Secondly, an epithelium may show the features of both subclinical papillomavirus infection and cervical intraepithelial neoplasia in the same area. Therefore, koilocytotic atypia, multinucleation and individual cell keratinization may occur in conjunction with the changes of cervical intraepithelial neoplasia (see Figs 12.26 and 12.27).

COLPOSCOPY

Colposcopically, subclinical papillomavirus lesions are best assessed after application of acetic acid (Fig. 12.28). The changes seen are: a shiny, snow-

Fig. 12.26 Combined cervical intraepithelial neoplasia and subclinical papillomavirus infection. The epithelium is showing all the features of cervical intraepithelial neoplasia, together with koilocytotic change of the superficial cells. H&E, x 32.

Fig. 12.27 Combined cervical intraepithelial neoplasia and subclinical papillomavirus infection. Superficial cells are showing prominent koilocytotic change, but in the lower two-thirds of the epithelium the features of CIN 3 are apparent. Note the tripolar mitotic figure. H&E, x 128.

Fig. 12.28 Subclinical papillomavirus infection. (a) Before application of acetic acid. **(b)** After application of acetic acid; the lesion is now obvious, with acetowhite change. **(c)** A biopsy confirms the diagnosis.

white lesion (Fig. 12.29); an irregular outline with jagged, angular or feathered margins (Fig. 12.30); and the presence of satellite lesions extending beyond the transformation zone (see Fig. 12.30).

Apart from acetowhite changes, subclinical papillomavirus infection is also assessed on the basis of vascular pattern of the lesion, and response to Lugol's iodine applied in the Schiller's test. Strong or partial uptake (Fig. 12.31) of the dye by the affected epithelium denotes glycogenation, which may be present in subclinical papillomavirus infection, compared to the negative staining response usually shown by significant degrees of cervical intraepithelial neoplasia.

Capillary patterns may be pronounced and could be confused with, or be difficult to differentiate from, the mosaic and punctation patterns characteristic of cervical intraepithelial neoplasia. Reid has described the vascular pattern of subclinical papillomavirus infection as consisting of uniform, fine vessels, loosely and randomly arranged, often as a horizontal mesh reminiscent of bizarre spider's webs. Non-dilated capillary loops may also run vertically towards the epithelial surface, with a uniform calibre

Fig. 12.30 Subclinical papillomavirus infection. Multifocal acetowhite lesions, irregular outline with angular shape and satellite lesions beyond the transformation zone. Note the encephaloid surface. Courtesy of Mr A Singer.

Fig. 12.29 Subclinical papillomavirus infection. A shiny, snow-white lesion is apparent.

Fig. 12.31 Cervical subclinical papillomavirus infection, extending beyond the transformation zone. (a) After application of acetic acid. **(b)** After application of Lugol's iodine, with partial uptake of dye by the lesion.

Fig. 12.32 Mixed condylomatous and subclinical papillomavirus infection lesions with cervical intraepithelial neoplasia on the cervix. The variety of vessel patterns for each lesion are clearly seen. Only multiple biopsies unravel the problem.

throughout their course (Fig. 12.32).

It is relatively difficult to distinguish between subclinical papillomavirus infection and cervical intra-epithelial neoplasia. Several groups of workers have attempted to produce scoring methods for establishing a differential diagnosis, with varying degrees of success. In routine practice, a final diagnosis will depend on histological assessment of the biopsy material, and the biopsy report will usually be the final arbiter. This is particularly true where a combination of both conditions is observed. In these circumstances, diagnosis will depend on the histology of biopsies from each area (see Fig. 12.32). Nevertheless, some degree of colposcopic assessment is required if punch biopsy is to be directed to the area of significant disease.

MANAGEMENT OF HUMAN PAPILLOMAVIRUS INFECTION

Should an attempt be made to treat all patients with human papillomavirus infection? Some authorities argue that all such cases should be treated because of the potentially carcinogenic effect of the virus, but this raises the question of how treatment should be carried out. Exophytic warts can be recognized and dealt with fairly simply. However, recent evidence shows that up to 80% of all women have HPV–16 DNA in cervical, vaginal and vulval epithelium. Therefore, how can HPV–16 DNA be eliminated from the entire lower genital tract, including the vulva?

Exophytic warts can be treated quite simply with podophyllin, trichloracetic acid, diathermy, cryocautery or laser. More recently, the use of local or systemic injection of Interferon has been reported. Exophytic warts on the vulva will be distressing to the patient, but when planning management the clinician should be aware that up to 10% of such lesions disappear within 12 months, without treatment.

Also, the colposcopist should remember that such warts may be associated with premalignant disease and should look specifically for any evidence of concurrent premalignancy: if present, it should be treated on its merits.

Cervical and vaginal warts are usually relatively easy to treat, as indeed are vulval warts when present in small numbers. However, it is difficult to eradicate very extensive exophytic warts which involve not only the vulva, but frequently the perineum and perianal areas. The colposcopist should look for evidence of intraepithelial neoplasia in these lesions, taking multiple biopsies before treatment is instituted. Laser vaporization (and, in the future, possibly Interferon) would seem to be the treatment of choice.

Frequently, further areas of exophytic warts will develop, but usually these are well localized and can be treated fairly simply.

If extensive warts are associated with intra-epithelial neoplasia, local treatment will often be ineffective and excision should be considered. Because of the large areas involved, especially if the perianal area is affected, the optimal treatment may be local excision of all affected tissue, immediately followed by skin grafting. Where the perianal area is involved, a preoperative colostomy may be necessary; this can be closed a few weeks postoperatively.

Since patients with subclinical papillomavirus lesions will have HPV1–16 DNA affecting the rest of the lower genital tract, it is debatable whether any form of treatment is likely to eradicate the disease. However, if subclinical papillomavirus is associated with intraepithelial neoplasia, a different approach will have to be considered. According to some authorities, CIN 1 is no more than a change induced by human papillomavirus, and indeed some workers have shown that up to 50% of lesions which feature human papillomavirus and CIN 1 will disappear spontaneously within 12 months. However, because other lesions progress, some authorities would advocate that all cases should be treated.

If, indeed, all of these lesions are treated, some women will undoubtedly receive unnecessary treatment. Therefore, if the colposcopist is certain that neither cytology, colposcopy nor histology raise the suspicion of invasive disease, consideration should be given to allowing the patient to proceed without treatment, provided that follow up can be assured. If follow up is doubtful, then a strong case can be made for treating at that particular time. However, human papillomavirus in association with CIN 3 should always be treated. As a general rule, if the colposcopist decides to treat human papillomavirus which is seen in association with cervical intraepithelial neoplasia, treatment should be exactly the same as for that degree of intraepithelial neoplasia. Since changes in the cervix are occasionally associated with changes in the vagina and vulva, a full inspection of the lower genital tract should always take place.

Subclinical papillomavirus infection of the vulva may present as 'burning vulva' syndrome. Colposcopic examination will show diagnostic microscopic changes, but before embarking on any form of treatment other causes of vulval burning and discomfort should be excluded. If treatment is thought necessary, superficial laser vulvectomy may be performed, but long term results of this procedure are proving disappointing.

HERPES SIMPLEX VIRUS

Histology

The histological appearances of a cervix infected with herpes simplex virus type 2 depend upon the stage of the disease. Biopsies are very rarely taken at an early stage of the disease, and therefore examples of the early stages are rarely available for study. Changes start in the parabasal cells of the squamous epithelium, with nuclear enlargement and development of multinucleate cells. The characteristic nuclear moulding without overlapping is a feature more easily appreciated in cytological preparations. Intranuclear inclusions are uncommon.

Vesicle formation and ulceration follows within approximately 36 hours. At this time, multinucleate giant cells may be identified at the edges of vesicles and in their bases, with a polymorphonuclear leucocyte infiltration and, often, basal cell hyperplasia of the adjacent epithelium. Once ulceration has occurred and secondary infection has supervened, changes are those of a non-specific, acute necrotizing cervicitis (Fig. 12.33). A very dense stromal infiltrate of acute and chronic inflammatory cells extends into the granulation tissue at the base of the ulcer.

Cytology

The cytological features of herpes simplex virus infection are easily recognized. The cells are characteristically large, with multiple nuclei which mould one another and show emargination of chromatin and empty nuclei (Fig. 12.34). Occasionally, large

Fig. 12.33 A cervical biopsy, showing acute necrotizing cervicitis in a woman with herpetic cervicitis. This is the same patient as shown in Fig. 12.39. Much of the surface epithelium is lost, apart from the right side of the biopsy. The stroma is densely infiltrated by acute inflammatory cells, with crumbling. An inflammatory exudate is present on the surface. H&E, x 12.8.

Fig. 12.34 Herpes simplex virus infection. A large, multinucleated cell, showing moulding of nuclei with emargination of chromatin. Papanicolaou stain, x 128.

Fig. 12.35 Herpes simples virus infection. Multinucleated cells, showing moulding of nuclei and large central inclusions. Papanicolaou stain, x 100.

Fig. 12.36 Herpes simplex virus infection. These cells are showing multinucleation, but the nuclear features are poorly defined as a result of necrosis. Papanicolaou stain, x 128.

intranuclear inclusions may be seen (Fig. 12.35), and this is believed to represent an early stage of infection.

If infection presents as a necrotizing cervicitis, the cells appear degenerate and necrotic, with only the ghosts of nuclei being barely visible (Fig. 12.36). With experience, the cytologist can recognize the characteristic nuclear features in mononuclear and binuclear cells (Fig. 12.37), and it is unlikely that cellular changes would be misinterpreted.

The inexperienced or unwary cytologist may confuse the appearances in the necrotic stage with invasive squamous cell carcinoma (also an area of clinical difficulty), or cervical intraepithelial neoplasia.

Colposcopy

Normally, the colposcopist will see herpetic changes only if the patient has vulval herpes and presents with vulval pain. Occasionally, the cervix will also be infected and should be examined, unless vulval pain is so severe that examination is impossible. If herpes is confined to the cervix, the patient will usually present with profuse vaginal discharge of sudden onset. Epithelial changes begin in the form of one or more vesicles which are of short duration and usually not visible. This stage is followed by ulceration within 24–36 hours (Fig. 12.38).

Sometimes the damage is so extensive that the areas of ulceration coalesce, and the cervix becomes the seat of one large ulcer with some of the appearances of invasive carcinoma (Figs 12.39 and 12.40).

Fig. 12.37 Herpes simplex virus infection. Several cells with single nuclei, showing emargination of chromatin and empty nuclei. These changes are identical to those seen in the nuclei of the characteristic, large, multinucleated cell on the left. Papanicolaou stain, x 128.

Fig. 12.38 Areas of early herpetic vesicles.

Fig. 12.39 Gross herpetic ulceration and acute inflammatory changes.

Fig. 12.40 Gross herpetic ulceration and acute inflammatory changes.

TRICHOMONIASIS

Cytology

This common protozoan infestation may be easily identified in cervical smears. The trichomonad appears as a small, blue-grey, poorly defined body with an elongated nucleus (Fig. 12.41); this must be identified in order to differentiate the protozoan from cell debris or mucus. The presence of the protozoan does not always give rise to active infection; some women are carriers, but on occasion the infection

Fig. 12.41 Specific infection. *Trichomonas vaginalis* is recognized by the elongated or slit nucleus in the pale blue, indistinct bodies (arrows). Papanicolaou stain, x 128.

Fig. 12.42 Specific infection. *Trichomonas vaginalis* is sometimes associated with the filamentous fungal organism *Leptothrix*, seen here as hair-like strands. Papanicolaou stain, x 128.

Fig. 12.43 Small red spots due to *Trichomonas* infection.

Fig. 12.44 *Trichomonas* changes following application of Lugol's iodine.

Fig. 12.45 'Strawberry' patches due to *Trichomonas* infection (a) Low power. **(b)** High power. **(c)** Following application of Lugol's iodine.

may be accompanied by a severe inflammatory reaction, with extensive cell necrosis.

Trichomonas can rarely be associated with *Leptothrix vaginalis*, a filamentous fungal organism which seems to be non-pathogenic (Fig. 12.42).

Colposcopy

The cervix appears red, due to hyperaemia occurring as a reaction to the trichomonas infection. Close examination shows that the cervix is covered by a multitude of tiny red dots, each of which is the tip of a dilated subepithelial capillary reaching almost to the surface (Fig. 12.43).

When this is compounded by the fact that some of the superficial squamous cells desquamate, relatively few cells remain between the tip of the capillary and surface; these cells are poorly glycogenated, and as a result application of Lugol's iodine shows a multitude of tiny non-staining areas (Fig. 12.44).

Occasionally, the cervix has a typical 'strawberry' appearance: large collections of capillaries are grouped together, to form a red spot which is visible to the naked eye (Fig. 12.45a,b). Subsequent application of Schiller's iodine will reveal that the epi-

thelium covering each red spot is non-glycogenated, and consequently the cervix has a speckled appearance due to the non-staining areas (Fig. 12.45c).

Candida albicans

The spores and hyphae of *Candida albicans* are easily identified, usually staining pink, although their colour can vary from almost colourless to pale blue or orange (Fig. 12.46).

Candidiasis may be frequently present without an associated inflammatory response, but in some instances degenerative cellular changes (see page 00) may be seen despite the lack of response.

Actinomyces israeli

Actinomyces is an anaerobic bacterium, most commonly seen as small aggregates (Fig. 12.47) in the cervical smears of women using intrauterine contraceptive devices, although occasionally large and multiple aggregates are present. Other bacteria and increased polymorphonuclear leucocytes are frequently seen in association with the *Actinomyces* organisms.

Fig. 12.46 Specific infection. The pink staining, spore bearing hyphae of *Candida albicans* can be seen overlying the central group of squamous cells. Papanicolaou stain, x 128.

Fig. 12.47 Specific infection. A small bacterial aggregate is shown, with a dense central area. The club-like filamentous projections, characteristic of *Actinomyces israeli*, can be clearly seen. Papanicolaou stain, x 128.

BACTERIAL INFECTIONS

Cervical smears often contain large numbers of bacteria which can be differentiated from the commensal *Lactobacillus*. If such bacteria are apparent in large numbers, both in the background of a smear and clustering on the surface of epithelial cells (Fig. 12.48), there is a very high probability that they represent a pathogenic infection. The presence of increased numbers of polymorphonuclear leucocytes (Fig. 12.49), histiocytes, occasionally lymphocytes and rarely plasma cells, increases this probability. The distinction between lactobacilli (Doederlein) and treatable bacterial infections is essential in terms of management (Fig. 12.50; see Chapter 5).

Although cytology cannot differentiate between the various bacterial infections, it is useful to alert the clinician to the presence of excessive numbers of bacteria which may render the smear unsatisfactory or give rise to problems of interpretation (Fig. 12.51). Microbiological screening, followed by appropriate treatment, may be advisable before another smear is taken.

Bacterial infections most commonly associated with cervicitis are *Chlamydia trachomatis*, bacterial vaginosis and *Neisseria gonorrhoeae*.

Follicular cervicitis

Follicular cervicitis may be associated with chlamydial infection; in cervical smears, large numbers of mature lymphocytes are characteristically seen (Fig. 12.52), often in wide streaks.

Once the pattern has been diagnosed, it is unlikely

Fig. 12.48 Bacterial infection. Large numbers of bacteria can be seen in the background and overlying the surface of squamous cells, partially obscuring the cellular detail. Papanicolaou stain, x 128.

Fig. 12.49 Bacterial infection. In this case, epithelial cells are completely obscured by polymorphonuclear leucocytes and lymphocytes with bacteria in the background. Papanicolaou stain, x 128.

Fig. 12.50 Bacterial infection. At first glance, this pattern appears similar to that seen in Fig. 12.48, but closer inspection shows that these bacteria are the rod-like Doederlein bacilli which are non-pathogenic. Papanicolaou stain, x 128.

Fig. 12.51 Degenerative inflammatory change. The squamous cells show nuclear enlargement with minimal chromatin change. These probably represent degenerative inflammatory change associated with bacterial infection or human papillomavirus infection. However, mild dyskaryosis cannot be confidently excluded.

to cause diagnostic problems in the future. However, the differential diagnosis between follicular cervicitis and cervical intraepithelial neoplasia may be difficult for the inexperienced cytologist. The possibility of a lymphoma or endometrial adenocarcinoma should also be considered in the diagnosis.

BORDERLINE CHANGES

The 'inflammatory' smear

The term 'inflammatory smear' is, regrettably, widely used in cytological reports. However, this term probably makes sense only to the cytologist responsible for such a report, as it is open to individual interpretation by the recipient clinician.

Cytologists need to give a great deal of thought to the identification of inflammatory responses in cervical smears, in relation to both cellular changes and background appearances, as well as to the way in which the patterns are combined. These features require careful analysis in an attempt to clarify and discriminate between unimportant and significant elements. Whilst some studies have suggested that women with 'inflammatory smear' reports harbour a high incidence of cytologically unrecognized cervical intraepithelial neoplasia, or even invasive disease, other studies have shown that up to 70% do not have significant cervical disease and therefore do not require colposcopy.

A conservative approach, identifying a treatable infection and repeating cytology after treatment, is probably all that is required in the majority of women in this category. Referral for colposcopy should be

Fig. 12.52 Follicular cervicitis. Numerous lymphocytes, often in large sheets or streaks, are seen when a lymphocytic follicle is scraped with the spatula during sampling. Papanicolaou stain, x 128.

reserved for the minority, who have recalcitrant infection or show persistent nuclear changes after a second or third smear.

Nuclear changes bordering on mild dyskaryosis

The introduction of this category was an attempt by the British Society for Clinical Cytology to assist in clarifying this area of uncertainty, both in terms of actual cell appearance and, more importantly, in linking the language and terminology used by cytologists (including the term 'inflammatory' smear) to a management policy. In this way, it was hoped that the small minority of women with cervical intraepithelial neoplasia or early invasive disease, whose smears fall into this category, would be followed up with cytology and referred after a short period for subsequent colposcopic management.

Adherence to the recommendations of the British Society for Clinical Cytology for colposcopic referral of patients should minimize the risk of not treating the proportion of women with significant disease (see Chapter 5). Cytologists have a responsibility to address the issue of 'inflammatory' smear, and should appreciate the importance of evaluating smears as being genuinely unsatisfactory for a reliable assessment. Equally, care must be exercised in identifying features of specific infections which indicate the appropriate treatment, and in critically evaluating cellular changes which do represent dyskaryosis or malignancy. A better understanding of the cause and effect of an inflammatory response in a cervical smear, together with a growing awareness of diagnostic pitfalls, should help to improve both cytological and clinical expertise in this area.

To some extent this has succeeded in abolishing many meaningless terms, but the arguments presented for 'inflammatory' smears still apply no clear cytological criteria, and therefore a great deal of subjectivity still remains. Furthermore, there is a temptation, especially for the inexperienced cytologist lacking in confidence, to use this category as a convenient 'dumping ground' without addressing the basic issues.

The biological potential of 'borderline' lesions at the bottom end of the scale of abnormality (which is the context in which this phrase is used here and is the generally accepted interpretation) is not known. With regard to their management, the consensus of opinion in Britain at present is to wait and see, rather than refer immediately for colposcopy. Since this may not resolve the situation and indeed may be detrimental to the well being of the woman concerned, referral is reserved for cases of persistent abnormality following a repeat smear at six months.

Organized, long term, case controlled studies are being set up to evaluate the significance of these lesions in terms of progression rates and optimal treatment regimens. In the meantime, strenuous attempts should be made by cytologists to agree on reproducible criteria, so that reliable management decisions can be taken.

Adherence to the recommendations of the British Society for Clinical Cytology for colposcopic referral of patients should minimize the risk of not treating the proportion of women with significant disease (see Chapter 5). Cytologists have a responsibility to address the issue of 'inflammatory' and borderline smears, and should appreciate the importance of evaluating smears as being genuinely unsatisfactory for a reliable assessment. Equally, care must be exercised in identifying features of specific infections which indicate the appropriate treatment, and in critically evaluating cellular changes which do represent dyskaryosis or malignancy. A better understanding of the cause and effect of an inflammatory response in a cervical smear, together with a growing awareness of diagnostic pitfalls, should help to improve both cytological and clinical expertise in this area.

13. *Management of Premalignant and Early Malignant Disease of the Cervix*

INTRODUCTION

The treatment of squamous cervical intraepithelial neoplasia, microinvasive carcinoma and glandular intraepithelial neoplasia (cervical glandular atypia and adenocarcinoma in situ) should be tailored to meet the needs of individual patients and particular lesions. The place of cone biopsy, hysterectomy and the more recent, conservative methods of local destruction in the current management of these lesions will be outlined. Newer approaches to improving the cone biopsy technique and efficiency, and reducing morbidity, will also be considered.

Glandular lesions will be considered separately, as they constitute a peculiar problem in that their natural history is less well understood, and occasionally they may involve the whole length of the endocervical canal.

KNIFE CONE BIOPSY

No woman with abnormal cervical cytology should be treated without prior colposcopic assessment. This applies to the primary surgical methods of management of cervical intraepithelial neoplasia, whether the choice of treatment is excision or ablation. It is logical to assume that the efficacy of a chosen method of treatment will be maximized when the topography of the individual lesion is known.

The terms 'cone biopsy' and 'conization' (see Chapter 9) are often used synonymously for a variety of surgical procedures, ranging from standardized biopsies with specially designed instruments, to large shaped cone/amputations of the cervix. Although originally cone biopsies were aimed at women with suspected early cancer, many of the early cones were used to treat benign cervical conditions. In 1938, Martzloff used cervical biopsy to detect the presence of premalignancy, which he described as 'carcinomatoid'.

Cone biopsy in the management of cervical intraepithelial neoplasia should always aim to achieve a combined diagnostic and therapeutic effect. Optimally, the tissue removed by the cone should include not only the abnormal epithelium, but also the whole transformation zone, including its caudal and cranial limits; that is, the original and new squamocolumnar junctions. Only in this way can a cone biopsy be deemed diagnostic and in turn therapeutic.

Indications for cone biopsy after colposcopy

In a majority of cases, colposcopic assessment in the presence of abnormal squamous cytology will allow accurate definition of the topography of the underlying lesion. Colposcopic findings will fall into one of the following categories (Fig. 13.1):
(a) The entire lesion and transformation zone will be visible, with or without the aid of an endocervical speculum.
(b) The lesion will be located within the transform-

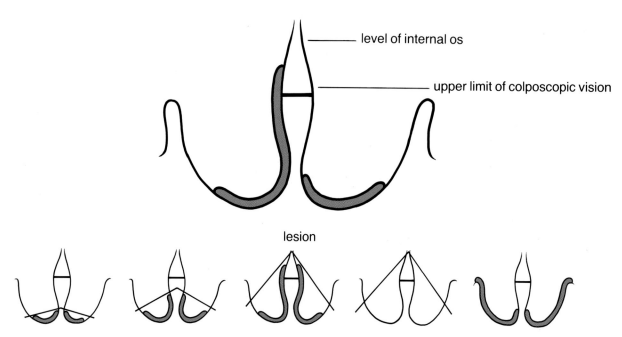

Fig. 13.1 Diagrammatic representation of classification of lesion topography after colposcopy. Lesion represented by bold line.

ation zone, but its endocervical limit will extend into the cervical canal, within or without colposcopic vision.

(c) Either (a) or (b), together with vaginal extension of the lesion.

(d) There is no lesion detectable to account for the abnormal cytology.

The examination may have revealed colposcopic appearances not only consistent with cervical intraepithelial neoplasia, but also raising a suspicion of breach of the basement membrane due to micro-invasive or frankly invasive carcinoma.

Moreover, in a minority of cases the primary cervical lesion may be part of multifocal intra-epithelial neoplastic change, involving the vagina, vulva or perianal region.

In all categories, a histological diagnosis is essential prior to treatment or as part of it if an excisional biopsy is involved. Where an expert colposcopy service is available, lesions in category (a) are suited to target or punch biopsy, followed by local destruction (see below). Lesions in category (b) carry a risk of hidden invasive disease in the non-visible portion lying within the endocervical canal.

The main indications for diagnostic cone biopsy after colposcopic assessment are as follows:

1. Lesion and/or transformation zone extend into the cervical canal, outside the range of colposcopic appraisal.
2. There is repeated abnormal cytology, suggestive of neoplasia in the absence of colposcopic abnormality.
3. Cytology suggests a graver lesion than that seen at colposcopy.
4. Any suggestion of invasive disease from cytology, colposcopy or directed biopsy.
5. There are atypical glandular cells in the index cytology, indicating the possibility of glandular intraepithelial neoplasia or adenocarcinoma.
6. Abnormal histology of endocervical curettings.

Where the entire transformation zone and the abnormality itself are visible, a small, colposcopically

tailored cone biopsy may be preferred to a locally destructive technique, as it carries the advantage of rendering all abnormal tissue available for histological study. In such cases, excision may be performed with the cold knife, carbon dioxide laser or large diathermy loop (LLETZ: large loop excision of the transformation zone; page 151).

Technique of knife cone biopsy

The optimal cone biopsy should remove the entire transformation zone. In all cases, colposcopy should allow accurate placing of the ectocervical circum-ferential incision, encompassing the lesion and all squamous epithelium containing evidence of underlying glandular activity, namely, surface gland openings or nabothian follicles. In most cases, the line of the old squamocolumnar junction may correspond to the outer edge of an acetowhite lesion. Sometimes, Schiller's test is used to define this ectocervical limit of an intraepithelial neoplastic lesion. However, it should be borne in mind that this test is associated with false positive and false negative correlations, as for example in cases of severe inflammation or oestrogen deficiency.

The major problem in cone biopsy is when the upper limit of the transformation zone or lesion is outside colposcopic vision, even with the aid of an endocervical speculum. In these circumstances, the actual length of the cervical canal requiring removal can only be a matter of conjecture.

Furthermore, cervical intraepithelial neoplasia may involve gland crypts to a depth of 4 mm on average below the surface of any aspect of the epithelium of the transformation zone. Therefore, if the apex of the cone is fashioned too narrowly, gland crypts affected by cervical intraepithelial neoplasia may be tran-sected, leaving residual disease in the stroma of the cone bed. In theory, this may be avoided by removal of a cylindrical block of tissue or a truncated cone (Fig. 13.2).

Fig. 13.2 (a) Possible sites for incomplete excision of cervical intraepithelial neoplasia. 1. Cone apex; 2. Glands in the stroma near the apex; 3. Ectocervical limit. **(b)** A truncated cone or cylinder should reduce problems at 2.

OPERATIVE TECHNIQUE

This is an inpatient procedure, requiring general anaesthesia. There is little to be gained by prolonged postoperative hospitalization, and most patients are able to leave hospital soon after surgery. A number of surgical variations have been described; the following is a common approach:

Preliminary ligation of the cervical branches of the uterine arteries is achieved by placing lateral sutures deep on each side in the substance of the cervix. Anterior and posterior sutures may also be used. The ectocervical circumferential incision is then made with a Beaver blade, ensuring several millimetres of clearance of the outer limit of the transformation zone.

Handling the surface epithelium must be avoided. Focal bleeding points are individually ligated, or diathermy is applied. No attempt is made to cover the cone bed by any form of suturing of the cut edges, thus minimizing the risk of burying residual abnormal epithelium where removal of the primary lesion is subsequently seen to be incomplete. Apart from the removal of the whole length of the cervical canal at biopsy, any decision regarding optimal cone length to ensure complete removal of the transformation zone on its endocervical aspect, where the new squamocolumnar junction lies out of sight in the canal, can only be arbitrary. This is unless more recent approaches to visualization are employed (see below).

If adequate haemostasis has not been achieved, it is best to avoid suturing. The cone bed may be packed with a 5 cm wide ribbon gauze, the tip of which has been soaked in proflavine in glycerine, or alternatively in Monsel's solution (see page 61). In a series of cone biopsies performed at the Northern General Hospital, Sheffield, Monsel's solution was the sole method of haemostasis, with no increase in haemorrhagic complications. The pack is removed on the following day, and the patient is discharged.

When the biopsy is completely removed without traumatizing the epithelium, an orientating marker suture may be placed in the stroma at the '12 o'clock' position (Fig. 13.3) for the benefit of the histopathologist, and the biopsy is placed in fixative in a container prelabelled with the patient's name (see Chapter 9).

IMPROVING TECHNIQUE AND EFFICACY, REDUCING MORBIDITY: NEW APPROACHES

In some cases where cervical intraepithelial neoplasia extends into the endocervical canal, beyond the limits of colposcopic vision even with the aid of an endocervical speculum, cone biopsy which removes the entire length of the canal may be required. However, as cervical intraepithelial neoplasia often does not extend far into the canal, this approach may be excessively radical, especially for patients in the reproductive age group.

Moreover, large cone biopsies are associated with increased short and long term complications. Appropriate, individually tailored cone biopsies could be performed in these patients, where it is possible to assess the extent of involvement of the canal by cervical intraepithelial neoplasia. This would increase the efficacy of the operation, and reduce morbidity.

MICROCOLPOHYSTEROSCOPIC ASSESSMENT OF THE CANAL

The Hamou microcolpohysteroscope (Storz, supplied by Rimmer Bros, London, UK) has been used to determine the extent of involvement of the endocervical canal in patients undergoing cone biopsy (Figs 13.4 and 13.5). With this technique, the epithelium is first stained with Waterman's blue ink which, in vivo, is taken up only by squamous cells. The blue stained epithelium is then visualized with the microcolpohysteroscope in the contact mode, with a 60-fold magnification and a resolution of 2 μm (Fig. 13.6).

When the highest point of the squamocolumnar junction within the canal is identified, its distance from the anatomical external os can be measured with the aid of a special sleeve with an expanded distal end (Fig. 13.7). Good correlation has been obtained between these measurements and subsequent histological assessment of the excised cone specimen. A considerable reduction in incomplete excision of neoplastic lesions is achieved, especially at the apex of the cone, when this method is employed to determine the appropriate cone length required in a given case.

Fig. 13.3 Cone biopsy specimen with orientating marker stitch at '12 o'clock'.

Fig. 13.4 Hamou microcolpohysteroscope, with additional metal sleeve to aid measurement of the distance to the squamocolumnar junction (see also Fig. 13.5). (Reproduced by kind permission of the *British Journal of Obstetrics and Gynaecology*.)

Fig. 13.5 Microcolpohysteroscopic measurement of the distance to the squamocolumnar junction. The junction is identified within the endocervical canal, and the metal sleeve is then pushed gently along the hysteroscope until the plastic washer is just resting on the cervix. Reproduced by kind permission of the *British Journal of Obstetrics and Gynaecology*.

Fig. 13.6 Microcolpohysteroscopy in contact mode. **(a)** Looped capillaries in a single villus; note the absence of blue stained squamous epithelium. **(b)** Normal squamous epithelium, top right; group of looped capillaries (indicating villi), bottom left; clear squamocolumnar junction visible.

(c) Dyskaryotic squamous epithelium on the right; villi immediately to the left, indicating true squamocolumnar junction. Reproduced by kind permission of *Colposcopy and Gynecologic Laser Surgery*.

Fig. 13.7 Metal sleeves for use in micro-colpohysteroscopic measurements: prototype (below) and commercially available type (Scaife endocervicometer; above).

149

LASER EXCISIONAL CONE BIOPSY

Knife excisional cone biopsy carries inherent morbidity, such as haemorrhage (primary and secondary) and cervical stenosis. One approach to minimizing these complications is to use the carbon dioxide laser, usually mounted on a colposcope, and with the micromanipulator as the cutting modality (Fig. 13.8a). Lateral cervical sutures may or may not be used to assist haemostasis.

Smaller excisional cones may be performed in this way on an outpatient basis, where a local anaesthetic is infiltrated under the cervical epithelium outside the lateral boundaries of the lesion (Fig. 13.8b). As a substitute for laser vaporization cone (see below), the excisional approach carries the advantage of preserving tissue for histopathological appraisal (Fig. 13.8c), which would be a safeguard against inadvertent vaporization of an unsuspected microinvasive lesion. In skilled hands, thermal artefact in the margins of the laser excised cone specimen does not interfere with histopathological interpretation.

Haemorrhage, infection and cervical stenosis are not reported as a problem, and the reformed squamo-columnar junction is visible at colposcopic follow up in a high percentage of cases; this is a clear advantage if residual disease is to be detected.

In addition, laser excision cone may be combined with more superficial vaporization of the extension of the main central lesion beyond the acquired transformation zone, even so far as the vaginal fornices. Usually, such an extensive procedure would require general anaesthesia, and it would be difficult to contemplate this with the cold knife.

The Nd:YAG laser, transmitted through a fine fibreoptic cable attached distally to an artificial sapphire tip which is contrived like a scalpel, has also been used as the cutting modality for excisional cones. This wavelength of laser light has a useful coagulative effect, and theoretically it should be associated with less intraoperative bleeding. However, the equipment is vastly expensive, safety aspects of its operation require meticulous care, and the method seems unlikely to find a place in routine conization except in the hands of a few enthusiasts.

LARGE LOOP EXCISION OF THE TRANSFORMATION ZONE

Excision of abnormal cervical epithelium by diathermy loop is based on an idea of Cartier who used a small diathermy loop to remove small pieces of cervical tissue for biopsy. The technique described by Prendeville involved a much larger loop which removed relatively large areas of cervical epithelium. The advantages of this procedure are outlined below:

1. Usually the procedure can be carried out on an outpatient basis, using local anaesthesia and a vasoconstrictor.
2. Bleeding is minimal.
3. Healing is rapid, with minimal fibrosis or stenosis.
4. The whole specimen can be sent for histological assessment, to discover any unsuspected invasive disease. This is an advantage, compared to the destructive methods which rely on a colposcopically directed biopsy or biopsies excluding areas of invasion before the destruction is carried out. However, this is rarely a problem for the experienced colposcopist, but for the less experienced the loop provides a very valuable safeguard against missing unsuspected invasion.
5. The histological specimen is processed in exactly the same way as a cone biopsy. Damage by the diathermy loop to the cut surface of the specimen is minimal and does not pose a problem to the pathologist.
6. The cost of the apparatus is relatively low; many operating theatres already possess diathermy equipment which would be suitable for this type of procedure (Fig. 13.9), and therefore the only expenditure would be that of the diathermy loops (Fig. 13.10).

Fig. 13.8 (a) Carbon dioxide laser and colposcope combination. (b) Carbon dioxide excisional cone in progress. This shows the manipulating hook on the cervix which is stained with Waterman's blue for preoperative micro-colpohysteroscopy. (c) Excised cone specimen, showing minimal thermal trauma and marker stitch in place.

7. The procedure can, if necessary, be carried out at the time of the first visit to a colposcopy clinic, thereby minimizing the number of visits which the patient has to make and the hospital has to provide.

The technique of diathermy loop excision is very simple and can be summarized as follows (Figs 13.11 and 13.12): The cervix is visualized using a standard laser adapted speculum, allowing smoke evacuation. The colposcopist delineates the area of abnormality to

Fig. 13.9 Diathermy/coagulator console, suitable for diathermy loop excision.

Fig. 13.10 Two sizes of diathermy loop for excision of the transformation zone, and a coagulation ball. Courtesy of Valleylab UK.

Fig. 13.11 Large loop excision of the transformation zone (LLETZ). (a) Cervix prior to LLETZ, with abnormal transformation zone highlighted with Lugol's iodine. (b) Completed LLETZ; large and deep cylindrical defect after four sweeps of the loop. (c) Loop biopsies reorientated and pinned to cork support.

(d) Histopathological preparation of loop-excised tissue, showing good clearance of glands to 1 cm depth. (e) Same cervix four months after treatment. Well healed cervix, with easily visible new squamocolumnar junction.

be removed. The local anaesthetic, combined with a vasoconstrictor, is injected at four points ('2, 5, 8 and 11 o'clock'). It usually takes about three minutes for the effects to take place; a useful endpoint is when the puncture marks, caused by the needle, stop bleeding. A loop is selected according to the size of the area to be excised. The loop is pushed into the normal tissue immediately lateral to the abnormality, at approximately '9 o'clock', and advanced to a depth of about 7–10 mm. The loop is then removed transversely from left to right, and exited on the other side of the cervix at a point lateral to the area to be excised. The base of the resulting crater is then coagulated by ball diathermy.

The wound is left open and the patient advised to avoid intercourse or the use of tampons and douches for three weeks. It is rarely necessary to use a pack or haemostatic agent.

Excision of a transformation zone too large to be accommodated by a single sweep of the largest available loop can be achieved with several systematic sweeps.

Hysterectomy and treatment of cervical intraepithelial neoplasia

Currently, routine hysterectomy in the primary management of cervical intraepithelial neoplasia is rarely practised. Indications for the procedure are mainly relative: coexisting benign gynaecological problems, such as dysfunctional uterine bleeding, fibroids, uterovaginal prolapse, or patient request for sterilization. Histological confirmation of neoplasia by punch or cone biopsy should be obtained prior to hysterectomy.

In selected cases, hysterectomy may be decided upon where the resection margins of a cone biopsy specimen show significant abnormality. Follow up cytology may indicate residual disease. However, even in such circumstances residual disease could be successfully treated with further cone biopsy or local destruction.

The lesion may extend on to the vaginal wall. Although a combined surgical and destructive technique may be used, hysterectomy may be the appropriate therapy in many cases. Colposcopy is essential to define the limits of the lesion and to establish the size of the vaginal cuff to be removed.

HYSTERECTOMY IN THE PRESENCE OF CERVICAL INTRAEPITHELIAL NEOPLASIA

Invasive carcinoma should first be excluded by colposcopically directed biopsy. The colposcopy allows clear characterization of the atypical transformation zone, which may extend on to the vaginal

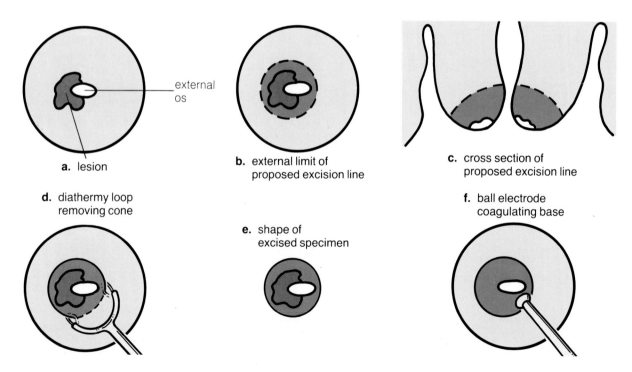

a. lesion

b. external limit of proposed excision line

c. cross section of proposed excision line

d. diathermy loop removing cone

e. shape of excised specimen

f. ball electrode coagulating base

Fig. 13.12 Diagrammatic representation of LLETZ. (a) Lesion in red. **(b)** External limit of proposed excision. **(c)** Depth and contour of tissue to be excised. **(d)** Excision in progress. **(e)** Excised specimen. **(f)** Ball electrode coagulating base.

vault. This has been reported in 5–10% of cases. Preoperative histological assessment of such vaginal changes should be obtained by biopsy. Although the epithelium may show acetowhite change or exhibit non-staining in Schiller's test, it is frequently histologically benign.

If the cone biopsy precedes the hysterectomy, it may be best to defer the operation for about six weeks, because of reported increased morbidity if the abdominal route is followed. If the vaginal route is chosen, the post-cone interval does not appear to matter. The route is a matter of personal choice or individual patient circumstances. In the majority of cases, simple hysterectomy is sufficient therapy, with or without removal of a cuff of vagina tailored to the individual lesion.

Several authors have emphasized the importance of the technique of closure of the vaginal vault. Mattress suturing of the vaginal edges (Fig. 13.13) and angles may result in any residual atypical epithelium being buried in the suture line, with colposcopic and cytological appraisal at follow up rendered difficult or impossible (Fig. 13.14).

While it is obviously important to ensure haemostasis, it is essential that the epithelium at the vault and angles after healing remain available for inspection. Invasive cancer has been reported to develop in these circumstances, where buried residual disease after hysterectomy remained.

METHODS OF LOCAL DESTRUCTION

The introduction of diagnostic colposcopy allows the topography of a lesion to be defined (see Fig. 13.1) and, where appropriate, the epithelium bearing the most severe change to be biopsied and the lesion to be histologically characterized. The technique has also contributed to improved cure rates of treatment by the traditional surgical approach of cone biopsy and hysterectomy. In addition, it has allowed the introduction of more conservative methods of treatment of cervical intraepithelial neoplasia, which are especially relevant in the younger women who constitute a significant proportion of presenting patients. Furthermore, these newer techniques offer the advantage of being predominantly outpatient procedures, and may be carried out under local anaesthesia.

By definition, cervical intraepithelial neoplasia is a local disease. It does not involve the underlying stroma or the lymphatics. The concept of applying a local biophysical method to destroy the epithelium is attractive, provided that the three-dimensional nature of these intraepithelial lesions is borne in mind (i.e. the degree of potential gland involvement by the process), as well as the fact that the entire transformation zone should be destroyed, as all its squamous epithelial cells may have been at risk of exposure to the carcinogenic process. In effect, these biophysical

Fig. 13.13 Commonly used closure of the vaginal vault at hysterectomy using the mattress technique. There is a danger of burying sheets or cords of intraepithelial cells.

Fig. 13.14 (a) Acetowhite change with punctation around and in the old suture dimple at the reconstructed vaginal angle following hysterectomy. **(b)** Photomicrograph of excised dimples in (a), showing residual vaginal intraepithelial neoplasia extending to 7 mm below the surface.

methods must seek to produce the equivalent of a small, colposcopically directed excisional cone.

Selection of patients

Over the years, strict selection criteria have evolved and should be observed (Table 13.1).

It is safer to manage patients or lesions not conforming to this check list by excisional cone biopsy (see above). It should be noted that almost four in five women over the age of 45 years will have a transformation zone out of sight inside the canal, and therefore are likely to require excisional cone.

Methods of local destruction

Methods of local destruction presently available for the treatment of cervical squamous premalignancy are radical electrocoagulation diathermy (the longest established method), cryotherapy, laser vaporization cone, and cold coagulation. As already mentioned, all of these methods seek to achieve the same effect, and it is imperative that the rigorous selection criteria are applied in each case. Two other methods of treatment (see above), although not locally destructive as such, are also finding favour: (a) the laser excisional cone, and (b) the large loop diathermy excision of the transformation zone. Both yield bulk tissue for histological examination, which is a clear advantage especially in the exclusion of unsuspected microinvasive disease. Both methods may be used as outpatient alternatives to local destruction of the transformation zone in selected cases.

Table 13.1 Selection criteria for local destruction
Assessment by skilled colposcopy
The whole transformation zone should be visible
Histopathology of punch biopsy from the most severe area of change should be available
No suspicion of invasive disease from cytology, colposcopy or histopathology
No suspicion of atypical glandular cells in the smear (i.e. suspected glandular intraepithelial neoplasia or carcinoma)

RADICAL ELECTROCOAGULATION DIATHERMY

Historically, this is the oldest of the local destructive techniques, developed by the Melbourne group under Chanen. Its main drawback is that its radicality demands general anaesthesia or regional block, usually on an inpatient or daycase basis, although recently Chanen has reported a successful feasibility study of the method carried out under local anaesthesia.

After induction of anaesthesia, the patient is examined in the lithotomy position and the colposcopy repeated to confirm the original findings. Chanen recommends dilatation and curettage at this stage. Dilatation should help to counteract any tendency to post-treatment stenosis. The cervix is painted with Lugol's iodine (Fig. 13.15a). The needle electrode is then used to outline the transformation zone, with a series of insertions 2–3 mm beyond the

Fig. 13.15 Radical electrocoagulation diathermy.
(a) Multifocal lesion highlighted with Lugol's iodine.
(b) Transformation zone after multiple applications of needle electrode to 8 mm.
(c) Procedure completed (after application of ball electrode).

iodine non-staining area. The entire transformation zone is then 'pepper-potted' with similar needle insertions at approximately 2 mm intervals (Fig. 13.15b). The needle is inserted to a depth of some 7–8 mm on each occasion, ensuring adequate destruction in depth to clear gland involvement.

On completion, the ball electrode is applied systematically to the entire surface of the circumscribed area (Fig. 13.15c). As considerable local heat is generated in the process, it is advisable to stop the procedure once or twice and douche the vagina and cervix with ice-cold saline.

It should be stressed that this radical destruction cannot be substituted by superficial diathermy or electrocautery, which will not guarantee a sufficiently deep destruction.

CRYOTHERAPY

Cryotherapy has also been used as a local destructive treatment for approximately two decades. The procedure is carried out on an outpatient basis, usually requiring no anaesthesia. The cervix is exposed, the earlier findings confirmed and the selected shape of cryoprobe applied and then freeze generated (Fig. 13.16a), until the resultant iceball extends 4–5 mm beyond the periphery of the probe (Fig. 13.16b). Usually, a three minute freeze followed by a five minute thaw and a further three minute freeze is recommended.

Reported cure rates with this method have been inferior to those of radical diathermy. In particular, the technique seems unsuitable for larger lesions (occupying half or more of the cervix) and high grade lesions (CIN 3). Another less significant drawback is the complaint of a watery discharge which may persist for several weeks after treatment.

CARBON DIOXIDE LASER VAPORIZATION CONE

Carbon dioxide laser light is especially well suited to local destruction of cervical intraepithelial neoplasia. With a wavelength of 10.6 μm, it is predominantly absorbed by tissue water, either intra- or extracellular, with little reflection or transmission through the tissue as forward scatter. By the use of appropriate power density at a focal point equivalent to that of the colposcope used to direct the beam, vaporization of tissue is achieved with a coagulative effect. An articulated arm brings the energy from the laser console to a precision micromanipulator which is attached to the front of the colposcope, and the carbon dioxide beam (invisible to the naked eye) is directed over the epithelial surface to be vaporized, with the aid of a visible red helium neon aiming beam.

The treatment is well tolerated, with a local anaesthetic injected subepithelially beyond the boundary of the lesion, and is performed under direct colposcopic control. Carbon dioxide laser vaporization offers the maximum degree of precision in tissue destruction, as the diameter of the beam is around 1.5–2 mm.

A cylinder of tissue is vaporized to the desired depth, which is usually 8–10 mm (Fig. 13.17). On completion, the depth of the crater can be measured with precision, which is not possible with any of the other methods of local destruction and is a clear advantage. Another positive feature of this technique is the ability to continue the vaporization process more superficially, to include any extension of the lesion on to the vaginal fornices. Healing is swift, with some epithelial covering present after three weeks. There is little or no necrotic debris, and therefore post-treatment discharge is minimal.

Fig. 13.16 Cryosurgical destruction of the transformation zone. (a) Probe applied and cryofreeze in progress. **(b)** Iceball effect following removal of probe upon completion.

Fig. 13.17 Cylindrical defect on cervix upon completion of carbon dioxide laser vaporization cone for cervical intraepithelial neoplasia.

COLD COAGULATION

The original cold coagulation apparatus was designed and used by Semm to treat benign lesions. The name 'cold coagulator' (Fig. 13.18a) is a misnomer, as the Teflon coated thermosounds are heated to a temperature of 100°C. Various sizes and shapes of sound or probe are available to suit the macro-anatomy of individual cervices and topography of lesions (Fig. 13.18b).

The procedure is performed on an outpatient basis, is well tolerated and usually requires no local anaesthesia, although some pelvic cramp-like discomfort may be experienced. The aim is to destroy the entire transformation zone (Fig. 13.19a), using overlapping areas of coagulation if required, and including the lower endocervix.

The average treatment time is 100 seconds, with each application of the probe lasting 20 seconds. When the probe is removed, a blistered appearance is noted and the superficial overlying epithelium is usually detached (Fig. 13.19b). As a result, it is virtually impossible to quantify the true depth of destruction achieved (Fig. 13.19c), which is a serious disadvantage of the method. In addition, there is postoperative discharge from the slough which is created by this process.

Results of local destruction

The success of locally destructive methods in 'curing' cervical intraepithelial neoplasia, based on relatively short term evidence of lack of residual or recurrent intraepithelial disease, seems to be very similar for the different techniques; it is in excess of 90%, and over 95% in some series. This compares favourably

Fig. 13.18 (a) Semm cold coagulator. (b) Various shapes of Teflon coated thermosounds for use with Semm cold coagulator.

Fig. 13.19 Local destruction of cervical intraepithelial neoplasia using Semm cold coagulator. (a) Pretreatment transformation zone; note the intrauterine contraceptive device in situ. **(b)** Coagulated transformation zone upon completion of treatment; note that the area is denuded of epithelium which has blistered off. **(c)** Same cervix after healing. Courtesy of Dr I D Duncan.

with the results of cold knife excisional biopsy and even simple hysterectomy. However, it would be a mistake to compare data from such dissimilar methods. Women subjected to treatment with local destruction represent a very carefully selected group. Most series report long term results of the traditional surgical excisional methods, dating from the days when all women and cervical lesions were similarly treated. Moreover, a 'cure' is considered real when there is long term evidence that treated patients did not subsequently develop invasive squamous cancer. Local destruction should be capable of destroying reliably and in depth, and lesions must be properly selected for this approach. With the methods to date, only radical diathermy (inserting the needle probe to a suitable depth), and laser vaporization cone (where the depth is actually measured) meet the former requirement. Errors will always be made in the selection process; undoubtedly, inappropriate local destruction of microinvasive lesions has accounted for some of the documented subsequent invasive cancers.

Reports are beginning to appear of invasive cancer following all local destructive methods. Fortunately, at present, the incidence seems no greater than for cone biopsy or even hysterectomy. Nevertheless, these cases underline the need for continuing vigilance, adherence to strict selection criteria and proper evaluation of new methods before they can be widely applied on a routine basis.

Where local destructive methods fail, as evidenced by cytological, colposcopic or histological suspicion of residual disease, there is a current view that the next step should be excision rather than further destruction. This trend is based on accumulating experience of repeat treatments and subsequent development of invasion.

In spite of these difficulties, it seems clear from studies to date that, with locally destructive methods, it is possible to retain the cervix and its function in a woman of reproductive age, without reducing the efficacy of treatment for cervical intraepithelial neoplasia.

MANAGEMENT OF MICROINVASIVE SQUAMOUS DISEASE

The difficulties over the histopathological aspects of stage Ia or microinvasive carcinoma of the cervix have already been discussed in Chapter 10. Microinvasive carcinomas are paradoxical in that they have all the hallmarks of invasive disease with breach of the basement membrane, and yet they are rarely associated with metastases.

In selecting women for less radical treatment, Coppleson holds that it is possible to recognize the odd case where spread may already have occurred by an integration of colposcopic observations into the pretreatment protocol. Before conservative treatment is employed, the following criteria should be met:
1. The lesion should not be colposcopically overt.
2. The colposcopic survey should be adequate.
3. The lesion should not present with atypical vessels, large tumour area or deep histological penetration and vascular space involvement.
4. Frank, crumbling tumour of the cervical canal should be excluded by endocervical curettage.

Conservative, simple hysterectomy, belonging to the less radical procedures, can be recommended in most cases. The ovaries need not be removed in the interests of curing the cancer. There is no strong case in favour of vaginal over abdominal approaches, although some gynaecologists may prefer the latter as it gives the opportunity of detecting any enlarged draining lymph nodes, although this is unlikely.

There is no indication for extending the operation to remove a cuff of vagina, except in the unusual case where extension of the cervical lesion on to the vaginal fornix has occurred, and this should have been recognized at the preoperative colposcopic assessment. In such a case, particular care must be taken over the histopathological measurements, as the large surface area may exclude the lesion from the category of microinvasion.

Whilst the above approach has been shown to be satisfactory, it would be of great disadvantage to the younger woman who still plans to start or increase her family. There is mounting evidence that, in these circumstances, a large cone biopsy, at least 2 cm long, may be safely considered as adequate therapy.

Alternatively, amputation of the cervix has been suggested, but this has no advantage over conization, provided that the latter has achieved eradication of disease, that is, the cone margins have been shown to be free of disease, both intraepithelial and invasive. In this group of women, the use of preconization microcolpohysteroscopic evaluation of the degree of canal involvement, with tailoring of the length of the cone to suit particular requirements, would be an advantage (see above).

MANAGEMENT OF ADENOCARCINOMA IN SITU AND CERVICAL GLANDULAR ATYPIA

The management of adenocarcinoma in situ and the less severe degrees of abnormality, cervical glandular atypia, presents as difficult a challenge to the clinician as does their detection and histological definition to the cytologist and pathologist. Undoubtedly, many cases of adenocarcinoma in situ and cervical glandular atypia are incidentally detected in cone biopsy specimens performed for suspected squamous neoplasia (Fig. 13.20). In addition, cytologists seem to have an increased awareness of exfoliated atypical glandular cells in screening smears.

Management

These premalignant lesions will be located in the field of cervical columnar epithelium. This includes columnar epithelium lying in the depths of crypts, or beneath squamous metaplastic epithelium in the glands of the transformation zone, and from the squamocolumnar junction to the upper limit of the endocervical canal at the internal os.

The abnormal epithelium may lie substantially beneath the surface. Thus, it is impossible to scrutinize colposcopically the entire target epithelium; indeed, any visible columnar epithelium is likely to represent a very small fraction of the whole.

Furthermore, even on rare occasions where a

Fig. 13.20 (a) Colposcopic findings in a case of squamous dyskaryosis in a smear. Note acetowhite change in the transformation zone (right), along with large hypertrophic villi with some showing acetowhite change and

contact bleeding (left). **(b)** Histopathology of the same cervix. Combination of cervical glandular atypia and intraepithelial neoplasia, showing as extension into the gland lined elsewhere by abnormal columnar layer.

Fig. 13.21 Colposcopy reveals large, hypertrophic, partly fused villi in the external os, with contact bleeding. Histopathology showed adenocarcinoma in situ with early invasion.

Fig. 13.22 Marked stenosis of the external os following cone biopsy. This renders endocervical cytology sampling difficult.

glandular colposcopic abnormality is identified (Fig. 13.21), it is not possible to confirm whether the whole problem is a single focus, as a multifocal disposition is also described.

It is clear that the only way of fully investigating the target epithelium is to have the entire length of the endocervical canal along with the transformation zone available for histological examination. This would involve a large cone biopsy removing the entire length of the canal, or alternatively a hysterectomy specimen, neither of which may always be appropriate. Therefore, the questions are raised as to whether a smaller cone biopsy which identifies a source lesion (or lesions) and whose excision margins are free of disease may be considered adequate treatment; or whether hysterectomy with excision of the whole cervical canal should be an obligatory next step.

The management dilemma hinges on our incomplete knowledge of the natural history of adenocarcinoma in situ and cervical glandular atypia; the inappropriateness of total extirpation of the uterus for younger women who undoubtedly are now presenting with the problem; and our uncertainty over the adequacy of cytology to identify ongoing exfoliation of abnormal glandular cells, especially if there are potential sampling difficulties (i.e. due to stenosis following an antecedent cone).

In the latter circumstances it would seem prudent to use one of the newer sampling devices, such as the Cytobursh or the Aylesbury spatula (see pages 50 and 51), for optimal collection of large numbers of columnar cells from the cervical canal, provided that this is readily accessible (see page 164).

Sometimes it may not be unreasonable to follow a conservative approach of observation without treatment, for example in the elderly or medically unfit patient. Also, where some additional gynaecological problem of a benign nature accompanies the adenocarcinoma in situ or cervical glandular atypia (such as fibroids, dysfunctional uterine bleeding or a request for sterilization), it may be wiser to proceed to hysterectomy, following the index cone biopsy which defined the premalignant nature of the disease and excluded invasion.

The same may apply to the older woman who has completed her family, although even in these circumstances removal of the uterus may be excessive. It is in relation to the younger woman that the real management dilemma arises. Here, the information from clinical studies is not available to allow clear recommendations. At present, the following seems a reasonable approach.

Regardless of age, in the presence of atypical glandular cells in the smear, a diagnostic cone biopsy is indicated, following colposcopy which, although unlikely to be helpful with the glandular lesion, may help to exclude any coincident cervical intraepithelial neoplasia. In the younger woman with a vested interest in future child bearing, this may be limited to removing 2 cm of the canal. It is unlikely that middle trimester abortion or preterm delivery in subsequent pregnancy are associated with this procedure. If the margins of the excision are free of the adenocarcinoma in situ or cervical glandular atypia, then no immediate further treatment is recommended, provided that follow up smears remain free of atypical glandular cells.

Where cone margins are involved, and the disease is apparently multifocal, hysterectomy would be indicated in the older woman, and seriously considered in the younger, although repeat cone biopsy may be a reasonable first option.

The mainstay of follow up is cytology, frequently in the first two years (four-monthly) and annually thereafter. After cone biopsy, both ectocervical and endocervical specimens are advisable (Fig. 13.22). Even after hysterectomy, vault smears at the same intervals are suggested. If atypical glandular cells reappear (see Fig. 11.24, page 120), further biopsy is indicated in the form of a repeat cone, hysterectomy, or full thickness biopsy from the vault if the uterus has already been removed.

Clarification of these difficult management issues will only come from appropriate clinical studies. These must be based on multicentre protocols so that sufficient numbers of cases are available for proper analysis. Finally, detection of a de novo primary lesion and of persistent or recurrent disease would be improved if a suitable cytological marker for the atypical glandular cell could be found in these selected cases.

14. Follow up after Treatment of Cervical Disease

REGENERATING/HEALING EPITHELIUM

Histological features

Re-epithelialization may take place in a variety of ways following treatment of cervical intraepithelial neoplasia, in spite of whether ablation or excision was the mode employed. Ideally, the treated surface will be covered by mature squamous epithelium within three weeks. Initially, this epithelium is of an important type, and consists of cells migrating from both edges of the treated area as well as from residual gland crypts (Fig. 14.1).

In an acid environment, differentiation and matur-ation into squamous epithelium will be encouraged. Quite often the maturation process of this new squamous epithelium will be impaired, and thus 'healing' epithelium, morphologically similar to im-mature squamous epithelium, will cover a small or large part of the treated area (Figs 14.2 and 14.3).

Consequently, the histopathologist is likely to encounter exactly the same difficulties in arriving at a differential diagnosis between healing epithelium and residual cervical intraepithelial neoplasia (see page 32), as in distinguishing between mature meta-plastic squamous epithelium and cervical intraepithe-lial neoplasia. This difficulty is compounded by the colposcopic impression that this epithelium, which is

Fig. 14.1 Cervix healing after laser vaporization cone.
Regeneration of squamous epithelium by metaplasia from columnar epithelium in gland crypts in the cone bed. PAS, x100.

Fig. 14.2 Healing epithelium following laser vaporization. The epithelium shows virtually no maturation; the appearances are very similar to those of immature squamous metaplasia. H&E, x32.

Fig. 14.3 Healing epithelium following laser vaporization. The nuclei are enlarged and show prominent nucleoli. They are uniform in shape, size and staining. Mitotic figures are infrequent and normal in configuration. H&E, x 128.

Fig. 14.4 Columnar epithelium growing far out on the ectocervix, following laser vaporization of a large area. H&E, x 32.

162

frequently acetowhite, represents residual disease (see below).

In circumstances that encourage an alkaline environment, the epithelium will frequently heal with islands of granulation on the surface. This is more likely to occur if very large areas are treated, where islands of villous, columnar, endocervical-type epithelium may be found on the ectocervix or in the vaginal fornices, amounting almost to an iatrogenic vaginal adenosis. Biopsy of these areas will show inflamed but otherwise normal 'endocervical' tissue (Fig. 14.4).

Cytological features

On most occasions, the cellular changes associated with regeneration and healing are easily recognized, since the features are similar to those of immature squamous metaplasia, and in most instances it may be difficult to make a cytological distinction (Fig. 14.5).

Healing following ablation of cervical intra-epithelial neoplasia, particularly if laser vaporization has been used, can be rapid. The cytologist is faced with difficulties in making a differential diagnosis between healing or regenerating epithelium and residual intraepithelial neoplasia (Fig. 14.6), as are the histopathologist and colposcopist.

The difficulties are compounded where the regenerative process is part of a chronic inflammatory response. This is probably one of the most significant areas where serious errors can be made in cytology, by failing to make the correct differential diagnosis between regenerative change and severe dyskaryosis or even invasive carcinoma (Fig. 14.7).

The cells may show nuclear enlargement with hyperchromasia and a prominent chromatin pattern. There is a homogeneous appearance to the cytoplasm, which appears blue or green in immature cells and pink in the more mature forms.

Fig. 14.5 Regeneration and healing. The cells in the centre are showing enlarged nuclei with some hyperchromasia but an even chromatin pattern and granular, pink staining cytoplasm, similar to the appearances seen in squamous metaplasia. Papanicolaou stain, x 128.

Fig. 14.6 Regeneration and healing. In this example, the nuclei are showing a marked hyperchromasia with coarse chromatin and dense blue-green cytoplasm. The distinction from dyskaryosis can be difficult. Papanicolaou stain, x 128.

Fig. 14.7 Regeneration and healing. The cells in the centre show a pale stained but irregular chromatin pattern. There is evidence of a chronic inflammatory response. Papanicolaou stain, x 128.

HEALING COMPLICATIONS

Stenosis

Cervical stenosis is reported after knife cone biopsy in about 1–4% of cases (Fig. 14.8). This is a much underrated complication, which may present as menstrual dysfunction or dysmenorrhoea. In severe cases, where occlusion of the canal is total (Fig. 14.9), amenorrhoea will result. This may be more common in women over 35 years of age, as a result of the greater endocervical involvement by cervical intraepithelial neoplasia in this group, necessitating a larger cone biopsy to effect cure.

Apart from the symptoms of stenosis, there is a further problem in following up the treated intraepithelial neoplasia: poor cell sampling may be obtained by the cytology spatula, and it may not even be possible to pass a fine endocervical brush if the os is too tight. The implications of not detecting residual disease are obvious, and if the os is completely sealed the patient may be at considerable potential risk in this respect.

In women of child bearing age, severe grades of stenosis may cause dystocia in subsequent pregnancy and labour. In older women, or where child bearing is complete, resorting to hysterectomy may be necessary in order to deal with the problem.

The traditional approach to the treatment of cervical stenosis involves vigorous dilatation of the cervix under general anaesthesia. However, this is often ineffective as stenosis tends to recur with time. More recently, the procedure of carbon dioxide laser endocervicectomy has been described, where the stenotic segment of the lower canal, often limited to only a few millimetres, is excised using the precision afforded by this modality. The results of this procedure seem fairly successful, as restenosis has been less frequently observed.

Stenosis has also been reported after local destruction for cervical intraepithelial neoplasia. It is recognized after cryotherapy and electrocoagulation diathermy (less than 1% of cases in Chanen's series), but is seen less after laser vaporization and excisional cones.

Data for cold coagulation do not suggest an excess of the complication, and information regarding stenosis after large loop excision of the transformation zone is not yet available. The problem in these circumstances may be managed as described following cone biopsy.

Squamocolumnar junction

Following treatment of cervical intraepithelial neoplasia by local destruction or excision, the squamocolumnar junction may (Fig. 14.10) or may not (Fig. 14.11) be visible and available for colposcopic and

Fig. 14.8 Cervix after cone biopsy suturing. Note the stenotic new external os.

Fig. 14.9 Total stenosis of the new external os after treatment.

Fig. 14.10 Cervix after cone biopsy. Adhesions have produced two tiny openings into the canal.

cytological assessment. The issue of whether a visible or invisible squamocolumnar junction is of clinical advantage or disadvantage is a subject of debate not as yet resolved by direct investigation. In the future, this issue may merit a prospective randomized trial, involving one or all treatment methods.

The desirability of a visible squamocolumnar junction after treatment is argued on the grounds of detecting residual or recurrent disease, either by colposcopy or cytology. Conversely, a squamocolumnar junction lying high into the endocervical canal will be outside the reach of whatever sexually transmitted agent causes the disease. This latter argument favours the role of endocervical cytology sampling devices. However, there is no scientific proof that visibility or invisibility of the squamocolumnar junction means that future development of invasive carcinoma is avoided.

Knife cone biopsy, with suturing of the cone bed for haemostasis, is more likely to be associated with a non-visible squamocolumnar junction after healing, and it may be that the suturing material is the main cause. This effect can be reduced if no sutures are used and haemostasis is achieved with a small pack with the end dipped in Monsel's solution (see page 61).

The carbon dioxide laser excisional and vaporization procedures have been shown to be associated with a greater visibility of the squamocolumnar junction (see Fig. 14.10). This may be partly because tissue is removed from the treated area at the time of the procedure, as opposed to leaving dead tissue to slough which is the case with some of the other methods.

However, laser excision, vaporization and loop methods have also been associated with endocervical tissue prolapse in a proportion of cases, observed at the first follow up examination (Fig. 14.12). This appearance is known as endocervical 'button', and could be taken as the ultimate exposure of the squamocolumnar junction after healing.

Laser techniques differ from the other destructive methods in that it is possible almost to 'sculpt' the end result, depending on the shape of defect produced in the cervix at the time of treatment. If laser vaporization or excision has been carried out high into the endocervical canal, the squamocolumnar junction will generally be invisible and the new external os will have a stenosed appearance. However, if after completion of the cone a shallow trench of approximately 1 mm in depth is vaporized around the ectocervical margin of the cone bed, the edge of the coned area will tend to evert, creating a 'button' effect on complete healing.

There have been anecdotal accounts of such endocervical prolapse being associated with recurrence of cervical intraepithelial neoplasia, but with no scientific proof. Over time, the exposed columnar villi

Fig. 14.11 Cervix at four months after laser vaporization cone. There is a visible squamocolumnar junction and metaplasia is proceeding in the exposed columnar epithelium.

Fig. 14.12 Cervix at four months following treatment. (a) After laser vaporization cone, showing pronounced endocervical button. **(b)** Same effect after large loop excision of the transformation zone.

covering the prolapse will undergo fusion, and later maturation of the squamous metaplastic process will ensue (Fig. 14.13).

The 'button' effect has also been observed after large loop excision of the transformation zone, which raises further speculation as to its true cause.

Other post-healing effects should be noted, as they may confuse the inexperienced clinician. After laser treatment, and also with some of the other locally destructive methods, subepithelial fibrosis may be marked; a pronounced white halo is seen around the new external os, before application of acetic acid (Fig. 14.14).

Furthermore, as part of the neovasculature response to healing, lines of punctate capillary loops may be seen radiating from the new external os (linear striations; Fig. 14.15). These should not be confused with punctation within residual disease. The healing vascular change will not usually be associated with acetowhite epithelium. Finally, lines of coarse ridges may be seen radiating from the new os, often with a hyperkeratotic appearance (Fig. 14.16).

Subsequent disease

None of the methods for treating cervical intraepithelial neoplasia offers an absolute cure rate, although most of them approximate this figure very closely, as gauged from long or short term data on follow up.

In this respect, and as regards the place of current, more conservative methods, the time honoured experience with knife cone biopsy and hysterectomy should not be forgotten. The ultimate test of 'cure' must lie in considerably long term follow up studies. For the surgical methods, these extend to not more than 25 years. In the literature, the risk of developing subsequent invasive squamous carcinoma of the cervix or vagina after treatment for cervical intraepithelial neoplasia by either surgical method is one case in several hundred. The data for radical electrodiathermy in the longest standing series now approach 20 years of follow up. The other methods are more recent, and their success rates still await the test of time.

For these reasons, patients must be carefully followed up to detect treatment failures (persistent or residual disease), as well as any recurrent disease of

Fig. 14.13 Cervix from a hysterectomy specimen. The patient had had a laser vaporization cone two years previously. Note mature squamous metaplastic epithelium over 'button'. No subsequent disease.

Fig. 14.14 Cervix at four months after laser vaporization cone. No application of acetic acid. **(a)** Note the dense white halo of subepithelial fibrosis. **(b)** White halo of subepithelial fibrosis together with radial ridges.

the cervix. The distinction between residual and recurrent disease is arbitrary, and of little relevance to the patient so long as it is detected and the chances of developing invasive disease in the future are kept to a minimum.

If it is felt that a distinction is required, then it is likely that cervical intraepithelial neoplasia discovered up to 12 months after treatment represents residual disease, and beyond that time the disease will be recurrent.

DETECTION OF SUBSEQUENT DISEASE

Both colposcopy and cytology are essential for the first and preferably the second visit. There is documented evidence that cytology following laser therapy may be negative in the presence of colposcopically overt residual disease which is confirmed at biopsy.

The first examination should not take place before four months postoperatively, as the ongoing healing process before this time may yield cells which are difficult to differentiate from dyskaryotic cells, and this epithelium may respond with acetowhite change (Fig. 14.17), causing further confusion.

Evidence of genuine residual or recurrent disease will usually carry the same colposcopic and cytological features as de novo lesions, most frequently revealed by acetowhite change (Fig. 14.19). Vascular patterns of punctation or mosaic may be present, the latter less commonly. Papillomavirus lesions in the healed area may be confused with cervical

Fig. 14.15 Neovasculature of healing, causing lines of punctate capillary loops. Four months after laser vaporization cone. No residual disease.

Fig. 14.16 Thick and hyperkeratotic ridges, caused by healing after laser vaporization cone.

Fig. 14.17 Acetowhite change in the region of the new squamocolumnar junction, four months after laser vaporization cone. Immature squamous epithelium on biopsy. No residual disease.

Fig. 14.18 Acetowhite epithelium on the edge of new external os and within the canal, four months after cone biopsy. Residual cervical intraepithelial neoplasia.

Fig. 14.19 Well demarcated acetowhite epithelium at the external os, four months after cone biopsy. CIN 2 with human papillomavirus changes.

intraepithelial neoplasia; biopsy will generally be necessary, offering a differential diagnosis.

These observations relate to subsequent disease located on the visible epithelium of the ectocervix or just inside the canal. Subsequent disease located high in the canal, for example at the healed apex of an excisional cone, cannot usually be seen through the colposcope, and will only be detected by a smear. The same may apply to deep seated disease after any of the destructive methods of treatment, especially if the new external os is, to some degree, stenotic.

TREATMENT OF SUBSEQUENT DISEASE

The treatment of cervical intraepithelial neoplasia appearing after therapy will depend on the nature of the lesion, its confirmed or suspected location, and the specific primary therapy which was used.

If subsequent disease appears after an excisional cone, it is best that repeat conization be performed. Where significant disease is suspected from cytology, with no colposcopically overt lesion identified, then an excisional cone would be prudent.

Occasionally, in the face of subsequent disease after a primary cone in the postmenopausal woman, further conization may be deemed technically impossible as the cervical remnant may be too small. In these circumstances, although harbouring the risk that unsuspected invasive disease may be encountered, hysterectomy may be the only feasible recourse.

Where subsequent disease arises after local destruction of cervical intraepithelial neoplasia, another attempt with this method may be permissible if the lesion is visible and confirmed on biopsy, and invasion has been excluded. In all cases considered for repeat local destruction, the lesion should be subjected to the same selection criteria used at the initial choice of the method.

Another problem is the continued exfoliation of dyskaryotic cells seen in vaginal vault smears, where hysterectomy had been the treatment of choice for cervical intraepithelial neoplasia: one of the main difficulties is to exclude buried vaginal intraepithelial neoplasia or invasive disease within the vault scar tissue. This question is addressed in Chapter 15.

POST-RADIATION CHANGES

Cytology

Treatment by radiotherapy is not appropriate for the majority of conditions dealt with in this book. However, occasionally smears will be taken from women who have had radiotherapy in the recent past, and it is relevant to mention at this point the cellular changes that may be seen.

Changes associated with radiation, which can be seen in non-neoplastic squamous epithelial cells, include multinucleation and bizarre forms, with gross cellular enlargement. Frequently, the nuclei are pale stained and have a characteristic wrinkled appearance (Fig. 14.20). It is important that the cytologist is alerted to the fact that radiation treatment had been employed, as these features can be confused with dyskaryosis or malignancy.

Fig. 14.20 Radiation changes. The cells are showing gross enlargement and variation in shape. The large cells appear bloated, and although the nuclei are enlarged the chromatin has a bland appearance. The cytoplasm is showing vacuolization characteristic of radiation change. Papanicolaou stain, x 128.

Fig. 14.21 Radiation changes. Note the prominent but regularly branching vessels.

Colposcopy

Following radiotherapy, the epithelium becomes relatively thin and atrophic, so that the subepithelial vessels may become clearly visible. The smaller vessels occasionally disappear, leaving only the larger vessels. The latter may be irregular and tortuous, and are sometimes dilated such that the inexperienced colposcopist may mistake them for vessels suggestive of invasive disease (Fig. 14.21). This misinterpretation is even more likely if the cytologist has already reported the presence of abnormal cells. Occasionally there may even be an avascular necrosis (Fig. 14.22).

TIMING OF VISITS

It is traditional for patients to be seen for a post-operative review approximately six weeks following gynaecological surgery, but after treatment for cervical intraepithelial neoplasia this can be counter-productive. If the patient is examined within a few weeks of treatment, regenerating cervical epithelium may have cytological and colposcopic features suggestive of persistent disease, whereas over a further few weeks these changes will disappear leaving a perfectly normal, mature squamous epithelium.

Another consideration is that visits to the clinic which are more frequent than necessary may cause concern and inconvenience to the patient, also generating extra work for the hospital and clinic staff. Many centres have shown that, for the average

Fig. 14.22 Post-radiation. Avascular necrosis is seen at the vaginal vault.

patient, there is nothing to be gained by following up too soon or too frequently.

However, if the first visit is delayed for a very long time, the colposcopist may miss persistent disease which requires further treatment. In the case of cervical intraepithelial neoplasia there is usually no major problem, but if the persistent disease is unsuspected invasive carcinoma or adenocarcinoma in situ, a delay could prove serious.

A number of centres arrange the first follow up visit at four to six months, or approximately one year after surgery, followed by annual smears. The subsequent frequency at which the patient is seen depends on local circumstances and will vary between one to three year intervals.

Ideally, at the time of follow up visits particular care must be taken to obtain cytology samples from the endocervical canal as well as from the ectocervix, especially if the pathologist has reported a suspicion of incomplete excision of the lesion.

Place of colposcopy

Combined colposcopic and cytological follow up will allow the colposcopist to detect persistent or recurrent disease with great accuracy. It has been estimated that a single cervical smear will prove to be a false negative in approximately 15–20% of cases, and the same applies to colposcopy. However, with the two techniques combined the false negative rate drops to 2–3%. Although it would seem ideal to combine cytology with colposcopy at each follow up visit, the sheer weight of numbers of patients attending most colposcopy clinics makes this an unattainable goal, and a compromise may have to be reached.

In the case of cervical intraepithelial neoplasia, a combined cytological and colposcopic assessment at four months (and afterwards perhaps once a year) can be followed by cytology alone, with the proviso that if an abnormal smear is obtained at any time in the future, colposcopic examination should be instigated. This follow up regimen also presupposes that the colposcopist can visualize the cervix adequately and, if necessary, take an endocervical sample.

If the original lesion is thought to have been incompletely excised, or where features of early stromal invasion or microinvasion are detected, a combined cytological and colposcopic assessment should be considered for the first five years.

15. Vaginal Intraepithelial Neoplasia

HISTOLOGY

Vaginal intraepithelial neoplasia (VAIN) is far less common than its cervical counterpart. It is most frequently seen in association with cervical intraepithelial neoplasia, sometimes as an extension of it. More usually, it is seen in the vaginal vault following hysterectomy for treatment of cervical intraepithelial neoplasia, where the line of excision has not been sufficiently wide to remove an unsuspected vaginal extension of it.

Less frequently, vaginal intraepithelial neoplasia may be found in the vagina at a site distant from the cervix; the cervix itself may be entirely normal.

The histological features (Figs 15.1–15.3) are very similar to those of cervical intraepithelial neoplasia. All possible variants are seen in the vagina, such as the changes of human papillomavirus infection. However, one important difference is the usual absence of gland crypts in the vagina, a significant feature when planning for local destructive treatment of vaginal intraepithelial neoplasia.

CYTOLOGY

The cytological features are similar to those of cervical intraepithelial neoplasia. The changes associated with human papillomavirus may also be seen, either alone or in combination with vaginal intraepithelial neoplasia (Figs 15.4–15.7).

COLPOSCOPY

When assessing a patient with a cervical intraepithelial lesion, the colposcopist must always consider whether the lesion extends beyond the cervix, into the vagina. Vaginal extension of cervical intraepithelial neoplasia will occur in approximately 1.5% of cases, and should be taken into consideration when planning treatment. Once vaginal extension is recognized, treatment will be straightforward. However, the presence of vaginal intraepithelial neoplasia following hysterectomy is a much more difficult clinical problem.

The colposcopic features of vaginal and cervical intraepithelial neoplasia are identical, and their interpretation usually presents little difficulty (Figs 15.8 and 15.9). In order to minimize the possibility of overlooking vaginal intraepithelial neoplasia, the

Fig. 15.1 VAIN 3. The appearances are identical to those of CIN 3, with loss of differentiation and nuclear abnormalities. H&E, x 32.

Fig. 15.2 VAIN 3. This example is showing irregular, bulky downgrowths and a little keratinization. H&E, x 32.

Fig. 15.3 VAIN 3. Slight papillomatosis and hyperkeratosis are seen. H&E, x 32.

Fig. 15.4 Vaginal intraepithelial neoplasia. Cells are showing mild, moderate and severe dyskaryosis. The nuclei are showing all the features of dyskaryotic change, except marked hyperchromasia. Papanicolaou stain, x 128.

Fig. 15.5 Vaginal intraepithelial neoplasia. This is a sheet of severely dyskaryotic cells, showing anisonucleosis and hyperchromasia. Numerous red blood cells are present. Papanicolaou stain, x 128.

Fig. 15.6 Vaginal intraepithelial neoplasia. A number of severely dyskaryotic nuclei are present, showing hyperchromasia, pleomorphism and irregularly clumped chromatin. Papanicolaou stain, x 128.

Fig. 15.7 Vaginal intraepithelial neoplasia. A well defined group of squamous cells is showing prominent koilocytotic change with binucleation; features associated with human papillomavirus infection. Papanicolaou stain, x 128.

Fig. 15.8 A coarse punctation pattern, extending from the cervix on to the posterior vaginal wall.

Fig. 15.9 Cervix exhibiting a mosaic pattern. The lesion is extending on to the right lateral vaginal wall, showing leucoplakia and gland openings. Biopsy revealed vaginal intraepithelial neoplasia.

inexperienced colposcopist is advised to use Lugol's iodine at the completion of every colposcopic assessment (Fig. 15.10).

It should also be borne in mind that the presence of vaginal intraepithelial neoplasia may be falsely suspected in a congenital transformation zone which frequently involves the vagina and has the colposcopic appearances of cervical intraepithelial neoplasia. Moreover, vaginal adenosis, whether or not associated with diethylstilboestrol in utero, undergoes physiological metaplasia which can be confused with vaginal intraepithelial neoplasia (see Fig. 19.7, page 214).

For these reasons, it is important to establish a histological diagnosis before attempting to remove what appears to be vaginal intraepithelial neoplasia.

Vaginal intraepithelial neoplasia following hysterectomy is usually suspected because of abnormal cytology, but when present it is usually easy to identify (Fig. 15.11). Care should be taken to inspect the vaginal angles where often a 'pocket' will be found; this pocket may be exposed using skin hooks or an endocervical speculum (Fig. 15.12).

Acetowhite epithelium, suggestive of vaginal intraepithelial neoplasia following hysterectomy, may sometimes be due to human papillomavirus infection (Fig. 15.13); it is, therefore, important that an adequate histological diagnosis is made before treatment is planned.

In the postmenopausal patient interpretation may be more difficult, and a six to eight week course of oral or intravaginal oestrogen could prove helpful.

Fig. 15.10 Vaginal intraepithelial neoplasia in the posterior vaginal fornix. This is in continuity with cervical intraepithelial neoplasia. **(a)** After application of acetic acid, mild acetowhite demarcated lesion is seen, with waxy leucoplakia. **(b)** Following Schiller's test.

Fig. 15.11 Residual vaginal intraepithelial neoplasia in the midpoint of the vaginal vault, after hysterectomy. **(a)** Following application of acetic acid. **(b)** Following application of Lugol's iodine, showing the biopsy site. **(c)** Biopsy showing VAIN 3.

MANAGEMENT

With uterus present

There are several treatment options to be followed, but each must be based on colposcopic assessment. These options involve methods of local destruction and surgical excision. When planning treatment by a destructive method, i.e. cryocautery, electrodiathermy or carbon dioxide laser, the gynaecologist should be aware of the proximity of the bladder, rectum and urethra in the operation field. In the postmenopausal patient the epithelium will usually be atrophic, and therefore it is advisable to prescribe a six week course of oestrogen before proceeding with local destructive methods.

Laser vaporization is probably the best mode of treatment. The operator must follow the same rules that apply in the local destruction of cervical intraepithelial neoplasia. It should also be remembered that vaginal epithelium has no crypts or clefts, and destruction to a depth of 2–3 mm will be perfectly adequate. Any associated cervical lesion can be treated on its own merits, by local destruction or excision.

In the case of associated menorrhagia, fibroid uterus or uterine prolapse, hysterectomy may be indicated, with removal of the appropriate cuff of vagina as determined by the colposcopic assessment of the lesion. Alternatively, it is possible to destroy the vaginal lesion first, and provided that at follow up the gynaecologist is satisfied that the vaginal lesion

Fig. 15.12 Residual vaginal intraepithelial neoplasia at the right vaginal angle, after hysterectomy.
(a) Acetowhite epithelium disappearing into the 'pocket' at right angle. **(b)** Vaginal angle pocket, opened with an endocervical speculum. **(c)** Biopsy from the lesion, confirming the presence of vaginal intraepithelial neoplasia with human papillomavirus change.

Fig. 15.13 Acetowhite epithelium suggestive of vaginal intraepithelial neoplasia following hysterectomy. This may often be due to human papillomavirus infection.

175

has been adequately dealt with, a simple hysterectomy may be performed.

Following hysterectomy

When planning treatment for vaginal intraepithelial neoplasia at the reconstructed vaginal vault following hysterectomy, the colposcopist should remember that the detected lesion is not a simple superficial lesion, as it is impossible to determine the amount of vaginal tissue remaining above the vault suture line (see Fig. 13.12, page 153). Failure to recognize this fact will often lead to inadequate treatment.

When the carbon dioxide laser was first introduced into gynaecology, it was thought that laser vaporization was the perfect way to treat these lesions. However, long term follow up showed that the failure rate was relatively high, and some patients subsequently presented with invasive carcinoma.

The reasons for this failure are quite obvious: the operator does not know how deep the laser destruction should be, being aware of the presence of other structures above, in front and behind the vaginal vault. Furthermore, vaporization must be preceded by an adequate biopsy, to exclude unsuspected invasive disease.

Alternatively, the colposcopically localized lesion may be surgically excised: small lesions can be adequately removed by local excision biopsy, lesions involving most of the vaginal vault by partial vaginectomy, and those involving most or all of the vagina by total vaginectomy (with or without reconstruction of an artificial vagina). However, the problem of not knowing how much vaginal tissue lies above the vaginal vault, especially in the lateral vaginal angles, still remains; any attempt to remove tissue deeply in this region carries the risk of damage to the bladder or ureters. Therefore, the abdominal approach may be considered more appropriate.

Because of these difficulties, treatment by radiotherapy has been advocated, offering excellent results. Prior to radiotherapy, the patient should have a colposcopically directed biopsy performed under general anaesthesia, aiming to exclude unsuspected invasive carcinoma. This is followed by insertion of one or two cylinders, each containing 15–20 mg of radium. The duration of insertion is between 72–100 hours, depending on the amount of radium used and the patient's tolerance to the procedure. The patient is discharged on the same day of treatment and instructed to start using a vaginal dilator daily, resuming normal sexual activity after four weeks. With this method, vaginal stenosis and dyspareunia are not usually a problem. In the premenopausal patient, ovarian function may cease, which is a clear disadvantage; in this case, oestrogen replacement therapy should be prescribed.

Intravaginal 5-fluorouracil cream has also been used in the treatment of supravaginal lesions. It is not well tolerated, and there have been mixed reports as to its efficacy in destroying these lesions.

MISCELLANEOUS VAGINAL LESIONS

Other than vaginal intraepithelial neoplasia, the most common vaginal lesions likely to be encountered are those induced by the human papillomavirus, discussed in Chapters 12 and 16.

A less common condition, occasionally seen at

Fig. 15.14 Endometriosis in vaginal fornices.
(a) Endometrioma; cervix above. **(b)** Endometriotic scarring in the left posterolateral fornix; cervix above and to the left.

Fig. 15.15 Recurrent malignant melanoma of the lower third of the vagina. Colposcopy has little to offer in this instance.

colposcopy, is endometriosis affecting the vaginal fornices (Fig. 15.14). Pigmented lesions of the vaginal epithelium are very uncommon, for instance clinically overt, pedunculated lesions of recurrent malignant melanoma, arising from the lower third of the vagina (Fig. 15.15). Colposcopy has little to add to their assessment.

16. Vulval Disease and Vulval Intraepithelial Neoplasia

CLASSIFICATION OF VULVAL DISEASE

The epithelial abnormalities of the vulva fall into three categories: the non-neoplastic epithelial disorders (previously known as dystrophies), papillomavirus infection and intraepithelial neoplasia (Table 16.1). In addition, because the vulva is an area of skin, general dermatological conditions, including psoriasis, ecsema, pemphigus, lichen simplex and lichen planus, must be borne in mind. However, a detailed account of these is beyond the scope of this book.

Non-neoplastic epithelial disorders

This is a group of skin conditions of unknown

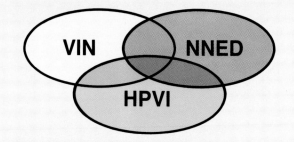

Table 16.1   Relationship between VIN, NNED and HPV

VIN   Vulva intraepithelial neoplasia
NNED Non-neoplastic epithelial disorders
HPVI Human papillomavirus infection

aetiology, and many terms have been used to describe them in the past. The current classification is shown in Table 16.2. Terms such as kraurosis vulvae, leucoplakia, leucoplakic vulvitis, atrophic leucoplakia, neurodermatitis, hyperplastic vulvitis and, most recently, dystrophy have been removed from the terminology of vulval disease; the term 'hyperplastic dystrophy' has been replaced by squamous hyperplasia.

Although the non-neoplastic epithelial disorders are presented in this classification as apparently distinct entities, it is probable that they are best thought of as a spectrum of disease, with the most hyperplastic forms at one end of the spectrum, and lichen sclerosus at the other.

Fig. 16.1 Squamous hyperplasia of the vulva. The thickening of the epidermis, with irregular prolongation of rete ridges, is apparent. The band-like, chronic inflammatory infiltrate hugging the lower surface of the epidermis is well shown. H&E, x 12.8.

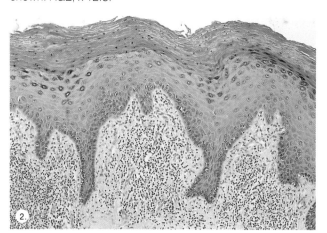

Fig. 16.3 Squamous hyperplasia of the vulva. An area showing slight atypia of the basal cells, with increased mitotic activity and some nuclear enlargement and hyperchromasia. H&E, x 128.

Fig. 16.2 Squamous hyperplasia of the vulva. Parakeratosis and a striking granular layer are seen. H&E, x 32.

Table 16.2 Non-neoplastic epithelial disorders of skin and mucosa of the vulva

1 Lichen sclerosus
   (lichen sclerosus et atrophicus)

2 Squamous cell hyperplasia
   (formerly hyperplastic dystrophy)

3 Other dermatoses

SQUAMOUS CELL HYPERPLASIA

This term characterizes the chronic vulval dermatosis which clinically has formerly been known as 'leucoplakia'. It is most commonly seen in postmenopausal women. The disease usually presents as vulval itching. The clinical appearances are of raised, white plaques on the vulva, which may involve both the labia majora and labial minora. Cracks and fissures appear, and from time to time red areas are seen.

The histological features are epithelial thickening with acanthosis, hyperkeratosis, parakeratosis and irregular prolongation of the rete ridges (Figs 16.1 and 16.2).

As leucoplakia is associated with hyperkeratosis, there is usually a prominent granular layer. The superficial dermis contains an infiltrate mainly of lymphocytes, but with some plasma cells and macrophages closely underneath the epidermis.

When atypia is present, it is seen as enlarged, hyperchromatic nuclei with chromatin clumping, mitotic figures and individual cell keratinization (Fig. 16.3).

LICHEN SCLEROSUS

This is a benign cutaneous disease of unknown aetiology, which is also encountered on the skin of the trunk, neck and extremities. It can affect any age group; the median age is just under 60 years, and approximately 60% of affected women are postmenopausal, although the condition may be seen in childhood.

The histological changes in lichen sclerosus of the vulva are the same as those seen at the extragenital sites. The most prominent feature is a broad zone of hyalinization and oedema in the papillary and reticular dermis (Fig. 16.4). The usual fibrillary pattern of the dermal collagen is lost, and elastic stains show a marked decrease in elastic fibres. Sometimes the oedema beneath the epidermis is so great that vesicles are formed.

The epidermis is thinned, with flattening of the rete ridges (Fig. 16.5), and there may be liquefactive degeneration of the basal layer. There is always hyperkeratosis, with the keratin layer often being thicker than the epidermis itself.

Fig. 16.4 Lichen sclerosus. The epidermis is markedly thinned, with 'flaky' hyperkeratosis. The hallmark of the condition is a clear, hyaline, oedematous band in the superficial dermis, beneath which there is an inflammatory infiltrate (rather sparse in this example). H&E, x 12.8.

Fig. 16.5 Lichen sclerosus. The epidermis is markedly thinned, and the skin appendage is compressed by the sclerotic superficial dermis. H&E, x 32.

MIXED EPITHELIAL DISORDERS

Squamous cell hyperplasia and lichen sclerosus may be mixed in two ways: first, it is not uncommon to encounter a vulval lesion which has adjacent areas of each type of abnormality. Secondly, an area may show some of the features of both forms of epithelial disorder, such that the epidermis is thickened, with hyperkeratosis and irregular elongation of the rete ridges, but with the superficial dermis showing the characteristic oedema and hyalinization of lichen sclerosus.

Papillomavirus infection

CONDYLOMA ACUMINATUM

The most striking feature of condyloma acuminatum is papillomatosis; in the absence of this feature, a diagnosis cannot be made. In addition, the lesion will show acanthosis, elongation of rete pegs, koilocytosis and, in some cases, a dermal inflammatory infiltrate (Fig. 16.6). Parakeratosis will very often be seen at the surface of the epithelium, and less frequently hyperkeratosis will be present.

Nuclear abnormalities are not apparent; the nuclei are uniform and show no hyperchromasia. Mitotic activity is often increased, but the mitotic figures are not abnormal.

SUBCLINICAL PAPILLOMAVIRUS INFECTION

The exophytic condyloma described above is not the only manifestation of papillomavirus infection of the vulva; 'flat warts' are also encountered. The term 'subclinical papillomavirus infection' is preferred, as it brings the terminology into line with that used for the cervix.

These lesions are not as frequently seen on the vulva as they are on the cervix. It seems that wart infection of the vulva is more usually associated with exophytic warts or intraepithelial neoplasia, whereas in the cervix the infection most commonly results in subclinical papillomavirus infection, or it is associated with intraepithelial neoplasia, with the exophytic condyloma being a relatively less common manifestation.

Vulval subclinical papillomavirus infection has the features of papillomavirus infection (see pages 129 and 130), koilocytosis being the most prominent. As in the cervix, this constellation of features may be seen in epithelium which also carries the features of intraepithelial neoplasia (Fig. 16.7).

Vulval intraepithelial neoplasia

For many years, the terminology of premalignant conditions of the vulva has been confused by the number and complexity of the terms used. In the last few years, the accepted terminology has been modified to bring the concept of preinvasive malignant disease of the vulva into line with that of the cervix. As a result, a system of nomenclature has evolved which uses the term 'vulval intraepithelial neoplasia' expressed as grades 1,2 and 3.

Even though this system of terminology is gaining general acceptance, it seems that application of the concept of a continuous spectrum of disease may be rather less appropriate in the vulva than it is in the cervix. The difficulty is compounded by the phenomenon of non-neoplastic epithelial disorders with which vulval intraepithelial neoplasia appears to

Fig. 16.6 Condyloma acuminatum, showing marked papillomatosis. Keratin is present on the surface, and a patchy, chronic inflammatory infiltrate is seen in the dermal core. H&E, x 12.8.

Fig. 16.7 VIN 3 with evidence of papillomavirus infection. The cells in the lower part of the epidermis are showing the features of VIN 3, but nearer the surface koilocytotic change and individual cell keratinization are prominent. H&E, x 32.

overlap at the mild end of its spectrum.

Moreover, many more cases of VIN 3 seem to be diagnosed than the less severe forms, which would not be expected if the disease was a spectrum of change, with the milder forms either progressing towards the more severe forms, or regressing (as is thought to happen in cervical intraepithelial neoplasia). However, this difference may lie in an inability to detect cases of lesser degrees of vulval intraepithelial neoplasia, which are usually asymptomatic.

HISTOLOGY

In general, the diagnosis of vulval intraepithelial neoplasia is histologically very similar to that of cervical intraepithelial neoplasia (Figs 16.7–16.12): it depends upon arrest of differentiation, maturation

Fig. 16.8 VIN 1. The epidermis is showing slight hyperkeratosis and some arrest of maturation. Nuclear enlargement and mitotic activity are slight. Koilocytotic change is present in this example. H&E, x 32.

Fig. 16.9 VIN 2. Mitotic activity and nuclear enlargement are in this example confined to the lower third of the epithelium. H&E, x 32.

Fig. 16.10 VIN 3. In this example there is considerable thickening of the epithelium, with striking papillomatosis. There is almost total arrest of maturation until the keratinized layer is reached. H&E, x 12.8.

Fig. 16.11 VIN 3. The cells of most of the thickness of the epithelium are showing nuclear enlargement, and mitotic activity is scattered throughout. H&E, x 32.

Fig. 16.12 VIN 3. Note the abnormal mitotic figure. H&E, x 32.

and stratification, nuclear abnormalities and mitotic activity (see Chapter 2).

As the grade of neoplasia advances, the proportion of epithelium showing differentiation decreases, the degree of nuclear pleomorphism increases, and mitotic figures are more numerous and are found at a higher level in the epithelium. Abnormal forms of mitotic figures are more common in the higher grades of disease. There is usually some degree of hyper-keratosis/parakeratosis, although this is not invariable.

The changes of vulval intraepithelial neoplasia may affect not only the surface epithelium; the pilo-sebaceous units can also be involved (Fig. 16.13). These may be as deep as 10 mm: a feature that must be taken into account when treatment is being planned. Involvement of skin appendages of the labia minora is very uncommon. A case of the duct of a sweat gland being affected by vulval intraepithelial neoplasia is illustrated in Fig. 16.14.

CYTOLOGY

Vulval cytology is limited mainly to those situations where cervical intraepithelial neoplasia is known to be present, or where colposcopic or clinical examination has identified a vulval lesion. The cytological features of vulval dyskaryosis are essentially the same as those described for cervical intraepithelial neoplasia (see Chapter 2).

However, vulval smears will contain predominantly keratinized squamous cells; indeed, some-

Fig. 16.13 VIN 3 affecting a pilosebaceous unit deep to the surface epithelium of the labium majus. H&E, x 12.8.

Fig. 16.14 VIN 3 affecting a sweat gland deep to the surface epithelium on the labium minus. Involvement of the skin appendage on the labium minus is uncommon. H&E, x 12.8.

Fig. 16.15 Invasive squamous cell carcinoma of the vulva. Large, bizarre, highly keratinized squamous cells are present, one of which is anucleate. Papanicolaou stain, x 128.

Fig. 16.16 VIN 3. The central group of cells are showing a keratinized cytoplasm. The nuclei are showing varying degrees of abnormality, amounting to severe dyskaryosis in three cells (arrows). Other cells are binucleate, suggesting the possibility of papillomavirus infection. Papanicolaou stain, x 128.

times it is the number and configuration of these highly keratinizing and bizarre-shaped, anucleate cells which will lead to the diagnosis (Fig. 16.15).

The nuclei of dyskaryotic and malignant cells may not appear hyperchromatic; on the contrary, they are frequently pale stained, and very few cells may be present (Fig. 16.16).

Occasionally, vulval smears from benign conditions are seen, and these are mainly composed of superficial squamous cells with some anucleate cells of normal shape and size. The features associated with herpes papillomavirus infection, already described, can sometimes be identified on vulval smears. In most cases, there are no reliable cytological criteria which can be applied to distinguish between VIN 3 and invasive squamous cell carcinoma.

COLPOSCOPY OF THE VULVA

Conditions other than vulval intraepithelial neoplasia and human papillomavirus-related disease should not be overlooked when a woman with vulval symptoms or a definite vulval lesion is referred for colposcopy. Where appropriate, the help of a colleague specializing in dermatology or genitourinary medicine should be sought (Figs 16.17 and 16.18).

Indeed, consideration should be given to setting up a specialist combined clinic for vulval disease, staffed by a colposcopist/gynaecologist, a dermatologist and even a histopathologist, all with a special interest, if the referral rate of vulval conditions to the colposcopy clinic is sufficiently large to justify it.

Colposcopy has not been found to be particularly useful in the examination of vulval lesions, compared with lesions of the vagina and cervix. For cervico-vaginal lesions, topography can be defined and some approximation of the degree of severity made, and the same approach may be employed to identify lesions on the vulva. This may be easier in the vestibule and on the medial aspects of the labia minora, where the epithelium is relatively thin (Fig. 16.19) or less keratinized.

However, keratinization interferes to a greater or lesser degree with the filter effect upon which grading colposcopic images on the cervix or vagina depends. Keratin is opaque, making evaluation of thickness of the affected epithelium difficult. Also, the vascular aberrations of punctation and mosaic are less commonly seen on the vulva, and if present they tend to be observed in lesions occupying the vestibule.

Fig. 16.17 Two common vulval conditions: (a) lichen sclerosus et atrophicus; (b) psoriasis. In these cases colposcopy has little or no place, and a dermatologist's opinion is essential.

Fig. 16.18 A rare dermatological condition of the vulva, which could be confused with cancer. Pemphigus vegetans of **(a)** the vulva and **(b)** umbilicus , showing similar change. In this case, colposcopy was of no diagnostic help.

Fig. 16.19 Vulva showing thin epithelial covering, with minimal keratinization over the vestibule and medial aspects of the labia minora.

Elsewhere, the vascular patterns may underlie but be obscured by keratinization. Ultimately, the colposcopist has to rely upon vulval biopsy to establish the true nature and severity of the lesion. Where vulval disease is multifocal, the colposcope may be invaluable in identifying the individual components, both for biopsy and treatment purposes.

Techniques of vulval colposcopy

The patient is examined in the lithotomy position. First, the vulva is inspected with the naked eye. Vulval intraepithelial neoplasia may appear as patches of white change, red or pigmented areas, or there may be an isolated or associated warty appearance. Using low power magnification (six-fold), the vulva is again scrutinized. Some of the obscuring effect of keratinization may be alleviated by thinly smearing a water soluble lubricant over areas of interest, to assist visualization of abnormal vessels. This is equivalent to the saline method for visualization of the cervix and vagina.

The junction between the glycogen bearing vaginal epithelium and keratin producing vulval epithelium is considered at high risk for intraepithelial neoplasia, and demands special attention. However, all areas of vulval epithelium should be systematically examined – the vestibule; urethral meatus; both aspects of the labia minora; the clitoris, prepuce and glans; the interlabial sulcus; the hair-bearing areas and perineal skin, concluding with the perianal skin and its mucocutaneous junction.

If a lubricant has been used, it should be removed with a dry gauze swab before using acetic acid on the vulva. This is best done by applying gauze swabs soaked in the 3–5% acetic acid, arranged so as to be in contact with the affected skin and left in place for approximately three minutes. After removing the swabs, a systematic scrutiny through the colposcope is repeated, using higher magnifications where appropriate. Areas of acetowhite change are noted.

Staining the epithelium with Toluidine blue is thought to help in the identification of certain lesions, especially if these are red in appearance due to lack of keratin. Excess blue dye is washed away by further application of acetic acid before an interpretation is made. Unfortunately, the dye is also taken up by fissures and excoriated skin. Not all colposcopists feel they can rely on this test, and some do not employ it at all.

It may also be wise to carry out a colposcopic examination of the anal canal, if the patient is tolerant of such examination. This can be performed with the aid of a proctoscope, and a device with a side-viewing slot is particularly useful. Direct visualization through the colposcope before and after application of acetic acid will be required.

If vulval intraepithelial neoplasia or human papillomavirus lesions are suspected, it is obligatory to proceed to a colposcopic examination of the cervix and vagina, if this has not already been done, including collection of a cervical smear for cytology.

Techniques of vulval biopsy

Histopathological confirmation of the nature and severity of lesions should be obtained from appropriate biopsy material. This may be by excision biopsy with a scalpel; by target biopsy (single or multiple), using the Keye's punch; or by wider excision of larger

Local infiltration in areas 1, 2, 3.

Fig. 16.20 Diagrammatic representation of full thickness excision biopsy of vulval lesion. This would be carried out under local anaesthesia.

Fig. 16.21 (a) Keye's punch for vulval biopsy.
(b) Magnified view of circular cutting edge (3–5 mm in diameter).

tracts of vulval skin. If required, closure with one or more sutures may be necessary, and depending on the circumstances the procedure is carried out under local or general anaesthesia, on an outpatient, day case or inpatient basis.

EXCISION BIOPSY

This type of biopsy is suitable where the lesion is small. A local anaesthetic block is injected subcutaneously, and the lesion is removed as an ellipse of full thickness skin, with several millimetres of clearance around the lesion (Fig. 16.20). A skin hook is preferable for handling the specimen in order to minimize crush artefact; this is introduced subcutaneously. Suturing with fine plain catgut is employed, as necessary.

DIRECTED BIOPSY WITH KEYE'S PUNCH

This standard dermatological biopsy instrument (Fig. 16.21) has a circular cutting edge, and a 3–5 mm diameter, and it may also be obtained as a disposable

for single use. It allows targeting of the biopsy from the centre of a lesion, and is also valuable where multiple biopsies are to be taken in multifocal disease (Fig. 16.22).

LARGE KNIFE BIOPSIES

In some cases, especially where the lesion is widespread, multifocal and confluent, a larger biopsy may be required and obtained under general anaesthesia. This procedure is designed to be excisional and curative.

The biopsy will be full thickness, ensuring that any skin appendage involvement by the intraepithelial neoplastic process is cleared (see above). Sometimes with extensive disease, it is not possible to be certain that invasion is not present without resorting to removal of a large tract of vulval skin. Closure with sutures will be necessary. This type of biopsy results in a variant of partial or total 'skinning' vulvectomy. In some cases, split skin grafting may also be required (see below).

Fig. 16.22 Technique of vulval biopsy using Keye's punch. (a) A solitary white lesion on the outer aspect of the (R) labium minus. **(b)** Punch applied with a circular motion. **(c)** Circular incision on removal of punch. **(d)** Biopsy bed after removal of specimen by undercutting with scalpel. **(e)** Haemostasis achieved with a single plain catgut suture.

VULVAL INTRAEPITHELIAL NEOPLASIA

As indicated above, intraepithelial neoplastic lesions of the vulva may be unifocal or multifocal. To the naked eye and through the colposcope they may appear white (leucoplakia; Fig. 16.23), red (Fig. 16.24), or pigmented (Fig. 16.25), and after a prolonged soak in acetic acid they may present by acetowhite change (Fig. 16.26).

Dense, keratinized areas may be a feature (Fig. 16.27), and a thin smear of lubricant may assist in visualizing an underlying abnormal vascular pattern, although this may not always be successful. Approximately 15% of intraepithelial neoplastic lesions are associated with previous or concurrent human papillomavirus infection, and an overlay of colposcopic features of the latter may be present as overt condylomatous change or subclinical papillomavirus infection. This may be easily confused with the raised, irregular surface of invasive disease, stressing the need for an appropriate biopsy in all cases.

As already discussed, the abnormal vascular patterns of punctation and mosaic or atypical vessels, so often a readily recognized feature of cervical and vaginal intraepithelial neoplasia or early invasive lesions at these sites, are not commonly seen in vulval lesions; this is partly due to the obscuring effect of keratin or indeed hyperkeratosis.

The naked eye appearance of the vulva in a case of chronic itching is seen in Fig. 16.27a. The clitoral area looks thickened, and there is an area of white change. At medium colposcopic magnification (Fig. 16.27b), with the aid of a lubricant and before application of acetic acid, the abnormal vascular pattern is obvious, along with dense white patches. These features are even more overt at higher colposcopic magnification

Fig. 16.23 Vulval intraepithelial neoplasia. A white lesion before application of acetic acid. A thick superficial keratin layer is seen.

Fig. 16.24 Vulva, before application of acetic acid, showing flat red lesions (VIN 3) on the left. On the right there is an adjacent, raised, irregular vascular lesion, with a linear area of thick white keratin (invasive squamous carcinoma).

Fig. 16.25 Vulval intraepithelial neoplasia. Pigmented lesions on the anterior vulva **(a)** and posterior vulva at fourchette **(b)**.

Fig. 16.26 Vulval intraepithelial neoplasia. A raised acetowhite lesion is seen on the outer aspect of labium minus and interlabial sulcus.

(Fig. 16.27c). A full thickness biopsy revealed an extensive VIN 3 with early invasion in several areas, as well as a thick, keratinized surface corresponding to the white patches. In Fig. 16.28, highly atypical vessels are seen at maximum colposcopic magnification, aided by lubrication only, in a case of recurrent invasive carcinoma of the vulva. Vessels are also seen running in 'corkscrew' fashion, parallel to the overlying epithelial surface, along with irregular dilatation producing a beading effect. It should be stressed that where an invasive element is suspected, as elsewhere in the lower genital tract, a full thickness biopsy is mandatory for a proper histopathological evaluation.

Management options

All cases of suspected vulval intraepithelial neoplasia must be diagnosed by biopsy, following the criteria elaborated above. The question of possible skin appendage involvement by the disease process must be taken into account in every case. Hair-bearing vulval skin may be a particular problem in this respect. Adequate biopsy should exclude or define this when present, ruling out microinvasive or frankly invasive disease. The preliminary colposcopy will also have helped in defining the topographical distribution of the lesion(s) on the surface.

Before outlining the available options for treatment, one further consideration must be borne in mind: with cervical intraepithelial neoplasia, some recent long term observations suggest that as many as one third of high grade lesions which continue to exfoliate dyskaryotic cells after the index biopsy may develop into invasive disease in time; however, the same data are not available for vulval intraepithelial neoplasia. In other words, at present our knowledge of

Fig. 16.27 (a) Naked eye view of clitoral VIN 3, with areas of microinvasion. (b) Medium colposcopic magnification, showing abnormal vascular pattern and white keratotic patches. Examination was with lubrication only, no application of acetic acid. **(c)** Vascular pattern seen at higher magnification.

Fig. 16.28 Recurrence of vulval carcinoma. Highly atypical vessels are seen with lubrication only; no application of acetic acid.

the natural history of vulval intraepithelial neoplasia and invasive squamous carcinoma of the vulva is lacking. Nevertheless, it seems likely that we are dealing with similar processes and possibly a similar aetiology.

Observation without treatment

The question may be asked, what happens to high grade vulval intraepithelial neoplasia if the lesions are simply observed? Some patients have been observed without therapy, and in one report five out of 50 (10%) cases of VIN 3 regressed spontaneously, even in the presence of aneuploidy in the lesion. Progression to invasive disease is also noted, although perhaps with a lesser frequency than might have been expected. However, care must be taken in drawing conclusions from such reports, in view of the relatively short periods of observation. More data are required in these areas, but clearly these will not

be forthcoming quickly if long term studies are required to deal with this problem. In the meantime, there may be occasions where observation without treatment may be justified, for example in the case of elderly and frail patients.

Surgery

The traditional treatment for vulval carcinoma in situ, as advocated by Knight, has been wide local excision. Many gynaecologists have preferred to remove the entire vulva, on the grounds that the disease was premalignant and often multifocal. This approach reflects the time when diagnostic colposcopy was not widely practised, and is akin to very large cone biopsy without colposcopic control for cervical intraepithelial neoplasia.

In addition, there is greater postoperative morbidity, and loss of the clitoris may render the patient anorgasmic; this may be a particularly important

Fig. 16.29 Extensive recurrent VIN 3. Previous treatment was by local excision, laser vaporization and 5-fluorouracil, but all methods failed. **(a)** Widespread red and pigmented lesions with areas of white change, partly due to scarring. **(b)** Preliminary vulval biopsy shows VIN 3 within the sweat gland ducts (above). **(c)** Preliminary biopsy shows hair shaft involvement by vulval intraepithelial neoplasia (dark staining haematoxylinophilic crescent on the left of shaft). **(d)** Superficial skinning vulvectomy completed, conserving the clitoris. **(e)** Fashioning split skin graft from donor site on the thigh. **(f)** Donor site on completion. **(g)** Completion of grafting on the vulvectomy bed.

consideration for the younger age groups in whom the disease seems to be more prevalent. Also, total vulvectomy is regarded as disfiguring by a number of treated women, irrespective of age.

These problems have led to the development of a more shallow excisional vulvectomy procedure, with conservation of the clitoris, if possible, and followed by split thickness skin grafting of the vulva using tissue from the thigh (Fig. 16.29).

Cryotherapy has also been advocated, and it may have a place in very small, isolated lesions without appendage involvement. However, it seems likely that such lesions will be more efficiently removed by excision biopsy in the first instance. Extensive freezing of large areas of vulval skin is likely to be followed by total sloughing, and painful and protracted healing, and is therefore not recommended.

Carbon dioxide laser

Carbon dioxide laser vaporization of the affected or all vulval skin in widespread disease has also been tried, with apparently good results following upon its success in the treatment of cervical and vaginal intraepithelial neoplasia. With this technique, intense, precisely controlled thermal destruction of the epithelium is possible under colposcopic control (Fig. 16.30). Reid has described four surgical planes of the vulval skin, and claims to be able to destroy the target tissue to the following depths (planes):
1. First plane: Surface epithelium.
2. Second plane: Dermal papillae.
3. Third plane: Pilosebaceous ducts.
4. Fourth plane: Depths of pilosebaceous unit.
It is feasible to achieve a depth of laser destruction to the first and fourth planes, as described. However, it is uncertain whether the same is possible for the intervening two planes. Healing of the vulva after superficial laser vulvectomy is protracted but with a satisfactory end result.

Vaporization to the depths of the entire pilosebaceous unit should not be undertaken without split skin grafting.

Chemotherapy

Topical 5-fluorouracil has also been used for vulval intraepithelial neoplasia. Overall response rates, as evidenced from published series, seem to be in the region of less than 50%. Local application is extended over six weeks, producing ulceration and sloughing. Pain may be intense, with significant non-compliance of patients. Remarkably, healing is associated with little scarring.

Treatment using sensitization to 2,4-dinitrochlorobenzene (DNCB) has also been described, producing ulceration followed by healing, as seen with 5-fluorouracil.

Treatment rationalization

Proper colposcopic and histopathological evaluation is a prerequisite for any form of treatment selected, with particular consideration of the need to exclude microinvasive and occult invasive disease and skin appendage involvement.

All destructive methods (cryotherapy, laser vaporization, 5-fluorouracil and DNCB) are limited by the disadvantage of not providing a total tissue specimen for histological appraisal. It is also doubtful and unproven whether 5-fluorouracil or DNCB sensitization can deal adequately with appendage disease. Although uncommon, early invasion may be present in some cases of apparent VIN 3, as is the case with CIN 3. If foci are recognized and adequately removed, prognosis is likely to be excellent.

Likewise, there are at present several studies quantitating the observed depth of appendage involvement by vulval intraepithelial neoplasia. Normal pilosebaceous units may project as deep as 10

Fig. 16.30 Vulval intraepithelial neoplasia. Superficial vulvectomy by carbon dioxide laser vaporization. **(a)** Before treatment, a red lesion is seen in the interlabial sulcus. **(b)** Vulva on completion of vaporization (Reid's second surgical plane).

mm below the skin surface, although it would seem unusual for the preneoplastic process to reach this depth.

For single or multiple lesions limited to the surface area, a wide local excision biopsy with or without suturing will probably suffice, both as treatment and for histopathological characterization. Lesions in the non-hair bearing skin of the vestibule and medial aspects of the labia minora, i.e. near the mucocutaneous junction, are suited to superficial carbon dioxide vaporization. The technique is also useful for small and multiple lesions in other parts of the vulva, provided that the histological criteria have been met.

Suspect invasion, biopsy proven appendage involvement, or very extensive disease are best dealt with by wide excision; in effect, this may represent hemivulvectomy or sometimes superficial excision of the whole vulva. In these circumstances, split skin grafting is indicated. The clitoris should not be removed unless it is clearly involved. Total vulvectomy carrying the dissection to deep planes is rarely indicated; the patient most likely would be elderly.

Irrespective of the treatment method applied, the recurrence rate of vulval intraepithelial neoplasia may be in the region of 15–20%, and close monitoring with colposcopy will be necessary. Any recurrent lesion must be biopsied and further treatment planned along the above lines. Follow up examination must exclude any de novo cervical, vaginal, urethral or anal lesions.

VULVAL PAPILLOMAVIRUS DISEASE

This can be subdivided into clinically overt lesions (condylomata acuminata and pigmented or non-pigmented papules), and subclinical disease, consisting of vestibular papillae, fused papillae and aceto-white epithelium. These will now be discussed with particular reference to colposcopic appearances; perianal and anal disease will also be addressed.

VULVAL CONDYLOMATA ACUMINATA

Condylomata acuminata of the vulva represent one level of a potentially multilevel sexually transmitted disease, with cervix, vagina and anal/perianal sites also likely to be involved.

Genital warts are now one of the most common sexually transmitted diseases, the reported prevalence having increased substantially in western countries over the last two decades. The majority of exophytic condylomata acuminata are induced by HPV–6 or HPV–11. More than 60% of sexual partners of infected individuals are reported to develop lesions after an incubation period of one to three months. Progression of genital warts to invasive cancer is well documented, although the relative risk is very low.

The naked eye appearance of condylomata at the vulval site is familiar (Fig. 16.31). Under higher magnification and after application of acetic acid, the agglomerated papilliferous acetowhite nature of the surface is obvious, each element containing an individual capillary loop (Fig. 16.32). Regardless of the apparently obvious naked eye or colposcopic diagnosis, a biopsy should be taken for confirmation.

Fig. 16.31 Vulval condylomata acuminata.

Fig. 16.32 Vulval condyloma after application of acetic acid. Marked acetowhite change and single capillary loop seen in individual fronds.

HUMAN PAPILLOMAVIRUS-INDUCED VULVAL PAPULES

Clinically overt, pigmented or non-pigmented papules may also be seen in human papillomavirus infection. These are raised, smooth and flat, and about 3–7 mm in diameter. The surface is often slightly glistening. Pigmentation may be present or absent. Less commonly, in negroid women, the papules may be associated with depigmentation. Lesions are frequently multiple and may coalesce. A biopsy would be necessary.

SUBCLINICAL HUMAN PAPILLOMAVIRUS INFECTION

This has been described in association with three types of lesion: vestibular papillae, fused papillae and acetowhite epithelium.

Vestibular papillae are multiple, small, spike-like projections of the vulval epithelium (Fig. 16.33), and as their name implies they are largely confined to the posterior fourchette, introitus and medial aspects of the labia minora. However, the external urethral meatus, the opening of Bartholin's gland ducts, minor vestibular gland ducts and Skene's glands are also reported as common sites.

The individual spike-like projections may occasionally appear to fuse or merge (Fig. 16.34), especially on the medial aspects of the labia minora, hence the name 'fused papillae'. This may result in a granular or velvety appearance, turning white after application of acetic acid. It has been claimed that these papilliferous lesions may be responsible for local pruritus or a burning sensation. For a time, an association between vestibular papillae, discrete or fused, and human papillomavirus was presumed. However, recent studies challenge this, and suggest that these appearances may be a variant of normal.

Finally, and less controversially, areas of vulval epithelium which turn white after application of acetic acid may be noted in otherwise apparently normal, flat vulval skin (Fig. 16.35). These acetowhite changes may affect any area, well keratinized or otherwise, hair-bearing or not. Biopsy will be required to give some indication of whether human papillomavirus or vulval intraepithelial neoplasia are implicated.

Fig. 16.33 Vestibular papillae. The multiple, small, spike-like projections are clearly seen.

Fig. 16.34 Fused papillae in the posterior lateral vestibule. These give rise to a naked eye velvety appearance.

Fig. 16.35 Acetowhite change associated with human papillomavirus infection. Vulva, over the perineal body posterior to fourchette.

PERIANAL AND ANAL LESIONS

Both intraepithelial neoplastic processes and human papillomavirus infection of the vulva may extend and involve the perianal region and anal canal. The appearance of such lesions is similar to those described above, under vulval disease. Firm lateral pressure on both buttocks may evert the anal canal to some degree, to reveal abnormality (Fig. 16.36).

However, proper exclusion or confirmation of disease in the anal canal requires the use of a proctoscope combined with a standard colposcopic technique, including application of acetic acid. If this is not tolerated in the outpatient setting, then daycase anaesthesia may be considered.

Any lesion identified should be biopsied using a standard colposcopic punch instrument with a small bite.

Fig. 16.36 Human papillomavirus-induced anal lesions. Patchy, fairly well defined acetowhite islands (subclinical papillomavirus infection) are seen, together with a small discrete condyloma.

Fig. 16.37 Gigantic juvenile vulval condylomata (HPV– 6/11 in)an 18 month-old. These were recurrent, despite several previous attempts to ablate using diathermy. **(a)** Immediately before treatment. **(b)** Immediately after combination treatment, involving initial excision of main bulk with electrodiathermy loop, followed by laser vaporization. **(c)** Three weeks after treatment; healing is seen to progress well. **(d)** Five weeks after treatment.

Treatment of human papillomavirus lesions

Vulval condylomata acuminata vary from small, readily treatable lesions to extensive superficial growths affecting substantial areas of skin, with a tendency to local recurrence which may become an almost intractable process.

Biophysical methods of eradication are usually employed, such as application of surface electro-diathermy, diathermy excision of larger masses, cryotherapy and carbon dioxide laser vaporization or excision (Fig. 16.37). Success in part relates to the fastidiousness with which similar lesions at the other common adjacent sites are identified and treated simultaneously, along with appropriate screening of the consort for human papillomavirus disease (Fig. 16.38).

For the moment, any recommendation as to the treatment of subclinical human papillomavirus lesions of the vulva must be given with caution. Our knowledge of the natural history, pathophysiology and progression potential of these lesions is incomplete. This includes our understanding of the precise role of human papillomavirus in the carcinogenesis of invasive squamous lesions of the anogenital tract.

Furthermore, there have been recent studies of the prevalence of human papillomavirus infection in the general and apparently well population, using the

Fig. 16.38 Human papillomavirus-induced papillae in the penile coronal sulcus.

new, highly sensitive polymerase chain reaction (PCR) technology for the identification of human papillomavirus DNA. These data suggest that an alarmingly high percentage of women and presumably their consorts may carry the virus.

Finally, there is little information to suggest that there is any reasonable hope of eradicating the virus from the entire anogenital epithelium by destroying subclinical papillomavirus infection with any of the available methods.

17. Oral Contraceptive Changes

HISTOLOGY

Microglandular endocervical hyperplasia

Microglandular endocervical hyperplasia (MEH; Figs 17.1–17.4) was first described in 1967. This is a combination of cellular changes in the endocervix, resulting from progestagenic influences on the epithelium. Although this condition is commonly seen in women taking the combined oral contraceptive pill and in pregnancy, it has also been reported in postmenopausal women.

Occasionally, microglandular endocervical hyperplasia is so florid that it presents as cervical polyps which are visible to the naked eye. However, more usually the cervix is macroscopically normal.

Multiple and apparently complex superficial cervical crypts are the most striking microscopical feature. Characteristically, the condition consists of numerous small glandular spaces lined by regular, cuboidal cells. The nuclei are uniform and vesicular, with occasional nucleoli. Mitotic figures may be present, but they are not found in every case. Sometimes vacuoles are prominent; these are often intracellular, although some are extracellular.

The 'microglandular' pattern of the lesion is produced by secondary gland formation, with budding of the endocervical crypts. Between the glandular epithelial elements there are cells which have the appearance of reserve cells, and immature squamous metaplastic elements can sometimes also be recognized. This finding suggests that microglandular endocervical hyperplasia may develop when conditions are right for squamous metaplasia, in the presence of a strong progestagenic stimulus. It is most important that the changes produced are not

Fig. 17.1 Microglandular endocervical hyperplasia. At low magnification, the surface of the cervix is seen to be polypoid. Reduplication of gland crypts is apparent near the surface. H&E, x 12.8.

Fig. 17.2 Microglandular endocervical hyperplasia. In addition to glandular reduplication, the more solid background of reserve cell hyperplasia is seen. This example also shows a moderate degree of inflammation. H&E, x 32.

Fig. 17.3 Microglandular endocervical hyperplasia. At higher magnification, 'signet ring' cells and pronounced subnuclear vacuolation are seen. H&E, x 128.

Fig. 17.4 Microglandular endocervical hyperplasia. In this example, maturing squamous metaplasia is mingled with glandular changes. H&E, x 32.

mistaken for malignancy.

Irregular nuclei and virtually absent mitotic figures are the most useful features for distinguishing the condition from carcinoma, but, as with so many other conditions, an awareness of its existence is the best safeguard for a correct diagnosis.

CYTOLOGY

Cervical smears from women taking oral contraceptives can vary considerably, ranging from smears of an almost atrophic pattern with mainly parabasal cells, to those showing a well oestrogenized pattern with predominantly superficial squamous cells.

However, a significant proportion of women, particularly those on high dose progestagen pills, present with unsatisfactory smears due to excessive

clumping and folding of the cells with large numbers of Doederlein bacilli (Fig. 17.5).

In the first instance, a repeat smear taken between the eighth and twelfth day of the cycle may prove satisfactory, but smears from some women in this group will always be unsatisfactory, irrespective of their timing within the menstrual cycle. It is therefore difficult to offer precise guidelines, and colposcopy may need to be considered in this small but significant group, as dyskaryosis may not be easy to identify.

Microglandular endocervical hyperplasia, although a well defined histological entity, is difficult to recognize and differentiate cytologically from endocervical cells of normal appearance, and reliable diagnostic features remain elusive.

COLPOSCOPY

At macroscopic examination, the cervix of a woman on combined oral contraception will often be red, friable, and covered with thick mucus, and the area around the external os may be showing an 'erosion'. At colposcopic examination, the cervix will often be enlarged because of generalized hyperaemia, such as occurs in early pregnancy. The squamous epithelium is seen to be unaltered in appearance, but changes are recognizable in the columnar epithelium. Individual columnar villi become enlarged and hyperaemic, and the apparent erosion represents nothing but enlargement and hyperaemia occurring in normal villi. In some cases these will increase to become almost polypoidal (Figs 17.6 and 17.7).

Sometimes enlargement of columnar epithelial villi

Fig. 17.5 Cytological appearances associated with oral contraception. Mainly intermediate cells are seen, with a few superficial squamous cells showing clumping and numerous Doederlein bacilli. Papanicolaou stain, x 128.

Fig. 17.6 Microglandular endocervical hyperplasia. In the lower part of the endocervical canal, some of the villi have become so enlarged that they have the appearance of small polyps. From Jordan and Singer, 1976, with permission.

Fig. 17.7 Clumped villi. Sometimes these can produce an irregular polypoidal mass which may appear quite abnormal at naked eye examination. From Jordan and Singer, 1976, with permission.

is such that columnar epithelium protrudes from the endocervical canal, resulting in eversion. Occasionally, this may be exaggerated by further eversion of the lower canal, following the insertion of a bivalve speculum. For these reasons, women are often incorrectly referred for treatment of an erosion which colposcopy shows to be perfectly normal epithelium.

18. Pregnancy

NORMAL CERVIX IN PREGNANCY

Three changes may be histologically identified in the cervix during pregnancy: decidual change, microglandular endocervical hyperplasia and Arias-Stella change.

Decidual change

Decidual change is an alteration in cervical tissue effected by the action of progestagens. Although usually regarded as a hormonal response of the endometrial stroma, it can also be seen affecting the superficial stroma of the cervix, as well as the lamina propria of the fallopian tubes, the surface of the ovaries, and the peritoneum.

Fig. 18.1 Decidual change in the cervix of a pregnant woman. A group of large, pale, decidualized stromal cells are present beneath the surface epithelium. H&E, x 32.

Microscopy shows features similar to decidual change at more familiar sites (Figs 18.1 and 18.2). The cells of the superficial cervical stroma are grossly enlarged and pale, with large, round nuclei and prominent nucleoli. The change is usually quite focal, affecting only a small area of the cervix. It may be situated on the endocervix or ectocervix. Occasionally, cells which are morphologically indistinguishable from endometrial granulocytes may be found amongst the enlarged stromal cells (Fig. 18.3).

Microglandular endocervical hyperplasia

This has been fully described in Chapter 17. There are no recorded differences between microglandular endocervical hyperplasia associated with pregnancy and that associated with oral contraception.

Arias-Stella change

As with decidual change, this phenomenon is more usually associated with the endometrium. However, very rarely, endocervical glands may show features of Arias-Stella change (Fig. 18.4). The most striking histological feature, in the endometrium as well as in the endocervix, is the presence of enlarged, hyperchromatic nuclei of irregular shape. This may or may not be accompanied by increased secretory activity. Distinction from glandular atypia may be difficult, but the presence of fairly abundant cytoplasm and absence of mitotic figures point towards a benign diagnosis.

Fig. 18.2 Decidual change. At higher magnification, the large, pale, decidualized stromal cells are seen. H&E, x 128.

Fig. 18.3 Decidual change. In addition to the decidualized stromal cells, this example also shows endometrial granulocytes (arrows). H&E, x 128.

CYTOLOGY IN PREGNANCY

The cervical smear pattern in normal pregnancy does not vary significantly from that seen in the normal secretory phase. On most occasions, the smear will be satisfactory for assessment, but in some instances the exaggerated progesterone effect may render the smear unsuitable, with excessive clumping and folding of the cells.

Navicular cells, since they are glycogenated intermediate squamous cells, are an indication of well marked progesterone response and should not be regarded as diagnostic or even suggestive of pregnancy.

A well marked oestrogen effect may suggest a deficient progesterone level, and the presence of endometrial cells in a cervical smear during pregnancy is an abnormal finding. Both observations should be reported.

Decidual change

On rare occasions, decidual change occurring in the cervix may give rise to large cells in the cervical smear. These have round, centrally located nuclei, sometimes with prominent nucleoli (Fig. 18.5). Since this finding is unusual, the decidual cells may be mistaken for dyskaryotic cells.

Arias-Stella change

Cytologically, the large cells with irregularly shaped and hyperchromatic nuclei associated with Arias-Stella change may be confused with dyskaryotic cells, particularly since this pattern is rarely seen in cervical smears.

ABNORMAL CERVIX IN PREGNANCY

Histology and cytology

The histological interpretation of material taken from a cervix during pregnancy is often said to be more difficult than that in the non-pregnant state. This is misleading because, once the changes described above are eliminated, there is no difference between the histological appearances of epithelial abnormalities in the pregnant and non-pregnant states.

Cytologically, the features associated with cervical intraepithelial neoplasia in pregnancy do not differ from those seen in the non-pregnant state (see Chapter 2).

GROSS PHYSIOLOGICAL CHANGES

In addition to the gross changes affecting the cervix and cervical epithelium during adolescence, pregnancy has a similar and major effect. At gross level, there are two changes: eversion of the endocervical canal, and gaping of the external os. The effect of these is exposure of previously protected columnar epithelium to the acid pH of the vaginal environment, and a reawakening of the process of squamous metaplasia. Eversion permits this by relocation of

Fig. 18.4 Arias-Stella change in the cervix. The appearances are similar to those frequently seen in the endometrium, with a slight increase in the complexity of the glands and a little increase in secretory activity. However, the hallmark of Arias-Stella change is the presence of enlarged and hyperchromatic nuclei. Mitotic figures are not seen. H&E, x 32.

Fig. 18.5 Cytology in pregnancy. The central group of cells have enlarged nuclei and abundant pale cytoplasm, characteristic of decidual change. Papanicolaou stain, x 128.

columnar epithelium to the vaginal aspect of the cervix, and gaping allows streaming of acidic vaginal secretions into the canal.

In the primigravid woman, eversion is the most important phenomenon, and its highest point is during the latter weeks of the first trimester. By contrast, gaping of the external os is an outstanding feature in the multigravida, and is evident from as early as twelve weeks of gestation.

In addition to these mechanical alterations, squamous metaplasia is observed (Fig. 18.6). Moreover, the exposed endocervical villi become large and hypertrophic, being partly responsible for the vascular appearance of the uterus. The uterus is also affected by alterations in the vascular tree itself, under the influence of pregnancy hormones. As a result, the cervix takes on its typical dusky bluish hue of pregnancy (Fig. 18.7). Glandular secretion increases, and the process of decidualization affects the stromal elements.

Finally, the effects of labour and vaginal delivery on the cervix and cervical epithelium must be considered. The passage of the fetus through a completely or incompletely dilated cervix produces substantial and easily recognizable injury to the epithelial and subepithelial tissues. These include:

1. True erosion or ulceration, with loss of surface epithelium.
2. Laceration, with extension of the tissue damage into the underlying stroma.
3. Bruising or ecchymosis.
4. Necrotic changes, colposcopically identified as yellow, featureless areas, usually associated with the edges of deeper lacerations. These lesions are obviously the direct result of trauma, and as such are more common in the primigravida after delivery, than in the multigravida.

Remarkably, healing is generally complete by approximately six weeks after delivery, at which time it is usual to find that the gross appearance and contour of the cervix bears little resemblance to its predelivery state.

As these active healing processes continue during the puerperium, it is usually best to defer further colposcopic assessment of women with abnormal cytology during pregnancy, until about three months post-delivery (see below); otherwise, confusing cytological and colposcopic appearances may be observed.

COLPOSCOPY OF THE NORMAL GRAVID CERVIX

The colposcopic appearances of physiological changes in the gravid cervix were presented in the 1970s by Singer, and the following account is based on that description.

In the primigravida in the early part of the first trimester, the cervix shows large areas of columnar epithelium with little evidence of squamous metaplasia. The latter process commences during the later weeks of the first trimester (see Fig. 18.7), coinciding with eversion. Very rapidly, islands of villous fusion occur, producing islands of immature squamous metaplasia.

This process becomes more active in the second trimester, and maturation occurs in the third trimester. Some metaplastic transformation also occurs within the canal, probably as a result of gaping of the external os.

In the multigravida, similar but more limited changes are observed. Metaplastic change tends to be a feature of the third trimester, accompanying

Fig. 18.6 Primigravida: cervix at 12 weeks of gestation. Early squamous metaplasia is seen, with fusion of villi.

Fig. 18.7 Primigravida: cervix at 16 weeks. Note the dusky blue background of the epithelium, due to underlying vascularity.

eversion. With gaping of the external os and streaming of acidic vaginal fluid into the canal, metaplastic change develops in the furrows or clefts within the canal.

Increased glandular activity is evidenced by profuse mucus secretion from gland openings which may be large and with pronounced rims (Fig. 18.8). Villi are large and hypertrophic, as seen in users of oral contraception. Vascularity produces a dusky bluish hue, and decidualization may present as 'doughnut' rims to the gland openings; in cases of extreme change, these may come to resemble 'mooncraters' (Fig. 18.9).

The eversion and gaping effects facilitate visualization of the new squamocolumnar junction. This is a useful and important consideration where colposcopy is performed in the presence of an abnormal smear.

COLPOSCOPY OF THE ABNORMAL CERVIX IN PREGNANCY

The indications for colposcopy in gravid women are more or less the same as those for non-gravid women. Namely:

1. **Dyskaryosis at cervical cytology:** Any woman with a positive cervical smear in pregnancy must receive a colposcopic assessment to determine the nature and severity of the underlying lesion.
2. **Human papillomavirus changes in the smear:** This indication may not be regarded by all gynaecologists as an absolute indication for colposcopy. However, it seems wise to attempt to define the exact nature of the lesion, as in the non-pregnant state, even though active treatment may not be contemplated. The association of human papillomavirus lesions with cervical intraepithelial neoplasia should not be forgotten (see page 132).
3. **Clinically suspicious cervix:** As in the non-pregnant state, clinical suspicion of possible underlying neoplasia, regardless of normal cytology, is an indication for colposcopy in pregnancy. Abnormality may have been observed through speculum examination, in cases of recurrent and otherwise unexplained bleeding at any stage of gestation. Alternatively, naked eye inspection of the cervix may have taken place during routine cervical cytology screening at an antenatal visit.

Colposcopic technique

During the first 16 weeks of gestation, the technique of colposcopy is basically the same as for the non-gravid woman. Both saline and acetic acid methods

Fig. 18.8 Multipara: cervix at 20 weeks of gestation. Large gland openings with umbilicated rims are seen.

Fig. 18.9 Gross decidualization of gland openings in pregnancy. (a) At low magnification. **(b)** At high magnification. Courtesy of Miss Rhona Stringer.

can be employed. In general, the appearances associated with underlying cervical intraepithelial neoplasia, invasive disease and the common human papillomavirus lesions are as would be expected.

Active squamous metaplasia in pregnancy, especially of the immature type, presents a difficulty. The condition may be typified by acetowhite change. Excessive mucus secretion may require a little more attention to interpret, prior to the formal examination.

Furthermore, the vascularity of the uterus may accentuate the patterns of mosaic, punctation and suspect atypical vessels, giving a colposcopist the impression that the existing lesions are of a higher grade than actual. However, because of the physiological eversion and gaping of the external os, the new squamocolumnar junction is often readily visible, rendering colposcopic examination satisfactory or complete in these instances (Fig. 18.10).

During the remaining 24 weeks of gestation, the saline and acetic acid methods may be employed. As pregnancy progresses, access to the cervix may become more difficult: the increasingly lax vaginal walls tend to collapse into the field of view, at times through the gaps in the sides of a bivalve speculum. Moreover, part of the fetus may present deep in the pelvis. The cervix may also be significantly displaced posteriorly towards the sacrum.

Despite these difficulties, it is extremely important that the entire examination is based on gentleness, as the tissues are easily traumatized. Even application of acetic acid needs care, and it requires a most delicate approach during pregnancy. In some colposcopy units, a spray bottle is used for applying the solution in pregnant and non-pregnant women. Sidewall retractors or ensheathing the bivalve speculum in a condom or one 'finger' from a rubber glove, with the end cut off, may help to overcome the problem of lax, bulging vaginal walls, thus facilitating this otherwise very difficult examination.

At this stage in pregnancy, punch biopsy is often accompanied by brisk bleeding, and therefore it should be undertaken only where absolutely necessary. If bleeding is encountered, simple pressure for a few minutes may control it. Monsel's solution, applied to the biopsy site even in pregnancy, almost never fails.

Management of abnormal cytology in pregnancy

A positive smear in the pregnant woman will always be a problem for subsequent management (Table 18.1). Before the advent of colposcopy, there was a tendency to rush to aggressive methods of diagnosis and treatment, namely knife cone biopsy. If the diagnosis is overt invasive disease, there is good reason for concern. However, this would be unusual, as such lesions are relatively rare and occur only in approximately one in 4000 pregnancies.

Cone biopsy in pregnancy is fraught with complications, including a higher incidence of primary and secondary haemorrhage. Increased perinatal mortality (stillbirth, preterm labour and abortion) has been attributed to this procedure, and is reported in 25–30% of cases. Furthermore, even after cone biopsy, the incidence of residual disease might remain in the order of 50%.

Despite these alarming statistics, two decades ago many gynaecologists would recommend this step in the management of a woman with a positive smear in pregnancy. However, colposcopy has created a much more conservative diagnostic approach, based on skilled, serial colposcopic appraisal in conjunction with parallel exfoliative cytology. Biopsy is thus minimized and limited to highly significant lesions where invasion cannot be otherwise excluded.

Fig. 18.10 Dusky blue cervix in pregnancy, with widespread acetowhite change. (a) Initial view, with the squamocolumnar junction not visible. **(b)** Minimal manipulation exposes the junction anteriorly.

Table 18.1   Suggested management protocol. Abnormal smear in pregnancy

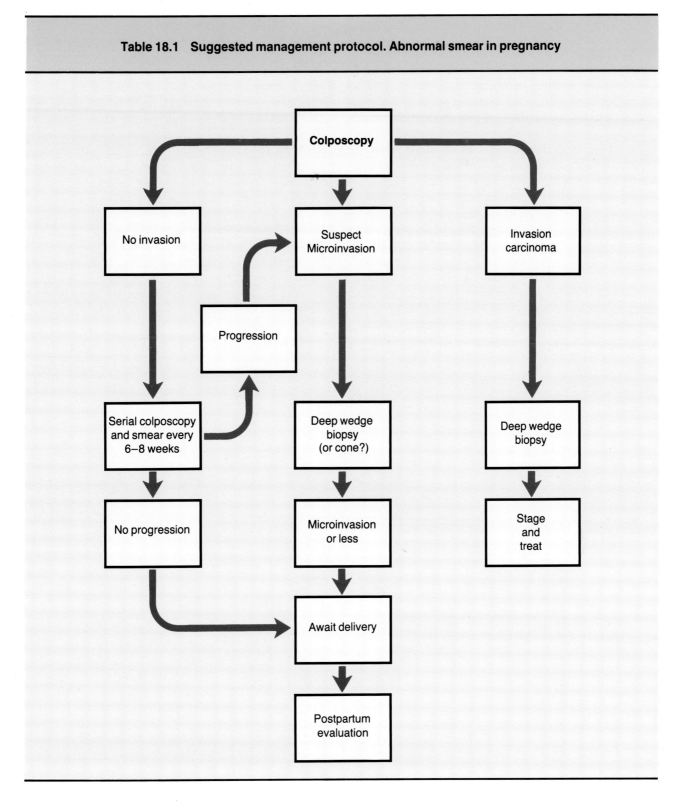

Management recommendations

At the outset it should be made clear that if, at any stage during pregnancy, there is colposcopic or cytological suspicion of microinvasive or frankly invasive disease, a large biopsy will be required for diagnosis; this will be either a colposcopically directed, deep wedge biopsy, or a cone biopsy. Obviously, either of these will be carried out under general anaesthesia.

MANAGEMENT OF LOW GRADE LESIONS

In this context, a low grade lesion will refer to subclinical papillomavirus infection, CIN 1 or CIN 2. Colposcopic examination should be carried out by an experienced colposcopist. Having established that the lesion falls into one of the above categories (Fig. 18.11; see Table 18.1), a confirmatory biopsy during pregnancy will usually be omitted, provided that the initial and repeat cervical smear reports are in broad agreement.

Colposcopy and cytology should then be repeated in each of the remaining trimesters, and again at approximately three months after delivery, when formal characterization of the lesion would be obtained by an appropriate biopsy. If necessary, treatment would also be selected. At any stage during this conservative management in pregnancy, a

Fig. 18.11 Cervix in pregnancy. This is a low grade acetowhite lesion with an irregular outline. Subclinical papillomavirus and CIN 1 are present.

biopsy might be indicated if the colposcopic impression or cytology suggest progression of the lesion.

Low grade lesions should not influence normal obstetric management of the patient, and in themselves are not an indication for elective Caesarean section. Proper colposcopic re-evaluation must be carried out at the postpartum examination. It is never appropriate to treat the cervix without this re-evaluation, as over the course of several months some low grade lesions may alter, either by regression or indeed progression.

MANAGEMENT OF HIGH GRADE LESIONS

High grade lesions imply CIN 3 (Figs 18.12–18.14). In addition, very large lesions of lesser grade would merit the same attention, as it may be more difficult to exclude progressive change occurring within a very large area.

Essentially, the management of these two groups is much the same as that for low grade lesions. However, as the risk of progression to microinvasive disease, although small, may be greater, re-examination both by colposcopy and cytology must be frequent, approximately every six weeks. The keystone of management is to observe for signs of microinvasion (see Fig. 18.15). These signs are the same as in the non-gravid state, and include the abnormal vascular patterns of markedly dilated vessels, vessels running horizontally in the epithelium, 'corkscrew' and 'comma' vessel configurations, and any significant increase in intercapillary distance.

It should be stressed that the increased vascularity of the gravid cervix tends to exaggerate vascular

Fig. 18.12 Cervix in pregnancy. This is a high grade lesion, with acetowhite change and a coarse mosaic pattern.

(a) At low magnification; note laxity of vaginal walls.
(b) At high magnification.

patterns, which may cause them to look worse than would be expected for the underlying lesion. Again, provided that the lesion remains intraepithelial, this conservative approach may be continued into the postpartum period and should not influence the obstetric management.

If concerns are expressed about possible breach of the basement membrane, then a large biopsy should not be delayed. This does not have to be a cone biopsy, as a large, deep (10 mm) wedge biopsy performed under general anaesthesia will often suffice to exclude microinvasion. The depth of any invasion present will help the histopathologist to differentiate between stage Ia and stage Ib disease, a point of considerable relevance to subsequent management.

MICROINVASIVE DISEASE IN PREGNANCY

The difficulty of establishing a diagnosis of microinvasion with certainty has already been alluded to, together with the need for a large biopsy in these circumstances to rule out frankly invasive carcinoma. Fortunately, evidence from the literature and local studies supports the view that progression of high grade lesions in pregnancy is an unusual event, and management of microinvasion in the gravid woman is uncommon. When it does occur, there are two considerations: maternal wellbeing and fetal welfare.

In the majority of cases, the maternal wellbeing will be paramount. For the fetus, the main concern will usually be whether it is sufficiently mature to survive outside the uterus; among other factors, this will depend on the gestational age and quality of available paediatric services. Currently it is possible to expect a reasonable chance of survival for a fetus of 24 or 26 weeks, if delivery is inevitable.

In the presence of an immature fetus, pregnancy may be allowed to continue if the diagnostic biopsy, especially a cone biopsy, shows complete excision of the lesion, provided that it comes within the criteria for microinvasion. Obviously, careful surveillance will be mandatory. There is probably no good reason for elective Caesarean delivery in cases of microinvasion in which the lesion has been completely removed by cone biopsy. Indeed, many gynaecological oncologists believe that Caesarean section need not be performed even in the presence of microinvasion.

At later periods of gestation, it is helpful if pregnancy can be allowed to continue until fetal lung maturity is reached. Again, it is not necessary to opt for Caeserean section.

Fig. 18.13 Cervix in pregnancy. This is a high grade lesion, with acetowhite epithelium and a mosaic pattern. Note the large hypertrophic villi, typical of pregnancy (below left).

Fig. 18.14 Cervix at 20 weeks of gestation. This is a mixed high grade lesion, with dense acetowhite epithelium on the left (CIN 3). The lesion on the right proved to be subclinical papillomavirus infection.

Fig. 18.15 Highly suspicious lesion in early pregnancy. CIN 3 with microinvasion.

209

FRANKLY INVASIVE CARCINOMA IN PREGNANCY

In general, pregnant women with a frankly invasive carcinoma of the cervix (Fig. 18.16) will usually be young, in the reproductive age group. Treatment is by radical hysterectomy with lymph node dissection, after referral to a gynaecological oncologist. Treatment of a pregnant woman should proceed without regard for the fetus, unless the lesion is discovered at a stage close to fetal viability, when a delay of a few weeks may be considered justifiable. In all cases, the views of a fully informed patient must be taken into consideration before any decisions are made.

Fig. 18.16 Atypical vascular pattern on clinically overt, raised, densely white, frankly invasive lesion in pregnancy.

19. Diethylstilboestrol Exposure

VAGINAL ADENOSIS

Vaginal adenosis is a benign condition in which normal columnar epithelium covers not only the cervix, but also part of the upper vagina. This condition reached prominence when it was reported that maternally ingested diethylstilboestrol exposure resulted in vaginal adenosis in approximately 90% of female offspring.

In addition to vaginal adenosis, other benign changes were recognized and have been collectively termed 'cervicovaginal deformities' (Table 19.1). These deformities tend to be called diethylstilboestrol changes, but similar changes can and do occur spontaneously, albeit uncommonly, in babies who have not been exposed to diethylstilboestrol in utero. These benign changes usually undergo spontaneous resolution over a period of time following transformation of adenosis to mature squamous epithelium by a process of metaplasia.

Interest developed in this particular cervicovaginal change, because of a theory in the early 1970s that these changes carried a high risk of producing clear cell adenocarcinoma of the vagina and/or cervix. It has been subsequently suggested that such patients have a higher incidence of premalignant squamous disease of the cervix.

The cervix and upper vagina may look peculiar, and in young women the changes can appear quite bizarre. In the past, these changes usually went unnoticed; this is due to fact that, as the young woman develops, the changes tend to disappear so that by the time she is first seen and assessed by a gynaecologist for some other reason, the macroscopically and colposcopically abnormal signs may have disappeared. The appearances of immature metaplasia on large areas of vaginal adenosis may be

Table 19.1 Relative incidence of cervicovaginal deformities n = 320

Cervicovaginal deformity	No. of patients	%
Type I cervix (circular sulcus on face of ectocervix)	117	36.5
Type II cervix (recessed area of perioral tissue)	22	6.9
Type III cervix (complete covering of ectocervix with endocervical epithelium)	22	6.9
Anterior cervical protuberance (smooth or rough)	46	14.4
Pseudopolyp	15	4.7

From: E. C. Sandberg (1976) Benign Cervical and Vaginal Changes associated with exposure to Stilbestrol in utero. *American Journal of Obstetrics and Gynecology*, **125**, 6, 777.

Fig. 19.1 Vaginal adenosis in a dethylstilboestrol exposed young woman. Courtesy of Mr J M Emens.

Fig. 19.2 Extensive areas of acetowhite epithelium undergoing metaplasia. Courtesy of Mr J M Emens.

worrying, because they share some of the features of premalignancy. Also, some of the irregularities noted on these cervices can give rise to concern, unless the colposcopist is aware of their significance.

Vaginal adenosis in a diethylstilboestrol exposed young woman is seen in Fig. 19.1. The cervix is covered by columnar epithelium which extends onto the posterior fornix and onto the posterior vaginal wall. Such areas eventually undergo metaplasia and produce large areas of acetowhite epithelium with some of the characteristics of CIN 1 (Fig. 19.2). It should be remembered that the incidence of vaginal extension of cervical intraepithelial neoplasia occurs in 1.5% of women with cervical intraepithelial neoplasia, who must have started their life with vaginal adenosis.

Multiple sulci on the ectocervix may also be seen (Fig. 19.3). The presence of an anterior cervical protuberance is often called a 'cock's comb', and this can be either smooth (Fig. 19.4) or rough (Fig. 19.5). The pseudopolyp formation is simply columnar epithelium confined to an area around the external os which is vascular and protuberant, giving the appearance of a large cervical polyp (Fig. 19.6).

Fig. 19.3 Multiple sulci on the ectocervix. Courtesy of Mr J M Emens.

Fig. 19.4 A smooth 'cock's comb'. Courtesy of Mr J M Emens.

Fig. 19.5 A rough 'cock's comb'. Courtesy of Mr J M Emens.

Fig. 19.6 A large pseudopolyp.

The cervix of a young woman exposed to diethylstilboestrol is seen in Fig. 19.7. The changes can be easily confused with extensive areas of cervical intraepithelial neoplasia.

On occasion, vaginal smears may be taken where the particular patient is known to have vaginal adenosis. These smears may show squamous metaplasia, together with glandular cells of endocervical type. It is important that a vaginal smear is taken with great care, to avoid contamination by metaplastic and glandular cells from the cervix.

It is important to remember that all of these changes can occur in non-diethylstilboestrol exposed young women, and if the colposcopist is examining women under the age of 20 these changes will be seen from time to time.

Fig. 19.7 Cervix of a diethylstilboestrol exposed young woman. (a) At low magnification, a smooth 'cock's comb' can be seen on the anterior lip. In the centre, there is a circular sulcus on the ectocervix. **(b)** Circular sulcus lateral to which there is acetowhite epithelium. **(c)** At high magnification, the acetowhite epithelium gives the appearance of fine punctation and mosaic patterns; the vessels are close together and signify immature metaplasia rather than cervical intraepithelial neoplasia. **(d)** The cervix and upper vagina are covered by non-glycogenated epithelium, clearly demarcating those areas which at one time in the woman's history had been columnar epithelium but at the time of examination was undergoing metaplastic change; in the present case the metaplastic change was complete. The epithelium was completely normal, and it is easy to see how this can be confused with cervical intraepithelial neoplasia.

20. Cervicography

INTRODUCTION

In 1981, Stafl introduced this new diagnostic method, cervicography, which combines the principles of colposcopy with a non-invasive photographic technique. It is claimed that this method adds less than one minute to a screening gynaecological examination.

Cervicography provides a permanent, objective photographic record of normal and abnormal cervical images, in colour. These may be taken by a doctor or suitably trained nurse, who need not be skilled in colposcopy. The only requirements are the ability to pass a speculum, visualize the cervix and be familiar with the photographic technique at a fairly basic level. The method also hinges on the response of the cervix to application of 3–5% aqueous acetic acid. After photographic development, the 35 mm image is projected onto a screen; the subsequent enlarged image is viewed and interpreted by an expert in colposcopy, who issues a report to the screener. The method was devised for use in conjunction with existing cervical smear screens, in the hope of producing a simplified combined screening, as opposed to cytology plus colposcopy, yet retaining the increased accuracy of the latter combination.

THE CERVISCOPE

The cervicographic camera is known as a 'Cerviscope' (National Testing Laboratories, St Louis, MO, USA) (Fig. 20.1). It is little more than an expensive, sophisticated 35 mm colour camera, with built-on

Fig. 20.1 The Cerviscope. Courtesy of National Testing Laboratories, St Louis, MO, USA.

flash, and fixed f-number, exposure time and focusing. This simplifies its use in relatively inexperienced hands, making it fairly 'foolproof' in terms of photography. The main operating features of the apparatus, which will be familiar to the average home photographer, are highlighted in Fig. 20.2. At the distal end of the arrangement, the examining light as well as the ring flash should be noted. The former allows adequate illumination of the cervix during focusing, which is done by moving the whole instrument to and fro. Thereafter, making the exposure demands no more than depressing the shutter release.

Fig. 20.2 Main operating features of the Cerviscope.

TECHNIQUE OF CERVICOGRAPHY

The procedure recommended for obtaining optimal cervicographs, once the cervix has been visualized with a standard bivalve speculum, is as follows:

1. As in colposcopy, the cervix should be wiped free of any blood or mucus, using a dry gauze swab.
2. Liberal application of 3–5% acetic acid to the cervix.
3. The cervix is viewed through the viewfinder of the Cerviscope, to ensure that the entire cervix is in the field. Further wiping of the cervix may be valuable at this stage, and any tenacious mucus may be displaced into the cervical canal using a cotton swab.
4. Liberal re-application of acetic acid.
5. Any extraneous examination light is extinguished, leaving the integral examining light in the Cerviscope as the sole source of illumination for the cervix. This step eliminates interference with the automatic exposure.
6. The instrument is aligned in the same axis as the vagina, and focus is on the cervix, moving the entire apparatus back and forth, as required.
7. The shutter release button on the pistol-grip is pressed smoothly and firmly.
8. After advancing the film, a second exposure should be taken (manufacturer's recommendation, if sending the film to them for processing and assessment by their professional evaluator).

Evaluating the images

After the film is developed, the slide (cervicogram; Fig. 20.3a) is projected at a standard magnification on to a screen. The projected image is claimed to be comparable to direct colposcopic visualization and resolution. Areas of acetowhite epithelium, vascular patterns and other such features should be identifiable (Fig. 20.3b). These images are interpreted by an experienced colposcopist and a report is issued. National Testing Laboratories offer this as part of their service, and the format of their reports is shown in Fig. 20.4.

There can be no question that this apparatus produces high grade photographs, and the technique can be mastered easily by non-colposcopists, provided that they are capable of visualizing the cervix using a bivalve speculum for the primary purpose of obtaining a screening cervical smear.

The main problems lie in the interpretation and evaluation of the projected images. These are limited to two dimensions, and for most colposcopists the lack of stereoscopic appreciation is restrictve, as is the fact that the cervicograph represents a single 'frame' in what, with a full colposcopic examination, is a dynamic imaging process.

Manipulation of the uterus, for detailed inspection of the vaginal fornices, for example, or determination of whether a given examination is unsatisfactory by the use of an endocervical speculum, is not possible. The limitations of interpretation will be obvious.

Fig. 20.3 (a) A typical cervicogram. This has been reproduced in actual size (inset). **(b)** Projected image of cervicogram.

Nevertheless, in conjunction with cervical cytology the technique is currently the subject of evaluation as an adjunct to screening. In one study involving just over 3000 women, cervicography was reported to detect almost five times more cases of cervical intraepithelial neoplasia than cytology alone. However, there was concern over the relatively high false positive rate for the cervicograms, necessitating referral for colposcopy, with associated emotional trauma.

The method has also been assessed for its value in detecting subclinical papillomavirus infection of the cervix, and is reported to be more sensitive than cytology alone.

It is unlikely that cervicography will ever replace colposcopy. If a lesion is detected by cervicography, expert colposcopic evaluation is necessary, along with appropriate colposcopically directed biopsy to define the lesion histopathologically. The final place of cervicography in our resources for cervical cancer prevention remains to be determined.

Cervicography result

☐ **Negative**

  ☐ The squamocolumnar junction and transformation zone are fully visible, no abnormal lesion present.

  ☐ The squamocolumnar junction is not fully visible but components of the transformation zone are visible on both lips, no abnormal lesion present.

☐ **Unsatisfactory**

  Components of the transformation zone are not visible on one or both lips. This can be due to:
  ☐ Previous cervical surgery   ☐ Other _____
  ☐ Physiological condition   _____
  ☐ Peri or postmenopausal   _____

☐ **Technically defective – retake cervigram!**

  ☐ Out of focus   ☐ Insufficient acetic acid or cervigram
  ☐ Overexposed   taken too late after acetic acid test
  ☐ Underexposed   ☐ Mucus or blood obscuring view
                          ☐ Speculum obscuring view
                          ☐ Vaginal wall obscuring view
                          ☐ Other _____
                              _____
                              _____

☐ **Suspicious**

  Abnormal lesion: Compatible with:
  ☐ acetowhite epithelium   ☐ immature squamous metaplasia
  ☐ punctation   ☐ mild dysplasia (CIN 1)
  ☐ mosaic   ☐ moderate dysplasia (CIN 2)
  ☐ atypical vessels   ☐ severe dysplasia (CIN 3)
  ☐ other _____   ☐ carcinoma in situ (CIN 3)
                                    ☐ microinvasive cancer
                                    ☐ invasive cancer
                                    ☐ papilloma, condyloma (HPV infection)
                                    ☐ other _____

Comments: _____
_____
_____
_____

Fig. 20.4 Cervicogram evaluation report. As used by professional evaluators of the National Testing Laboratories. Courtesy of National Testing Laboratories, St Louis, MO, USA.

21. *Planning and Management of Colposcopy and Outpatient Treatment Services*

INTRODUCTION

All district health authorities in England and Wales have been instructed to introduce computerized call and recall schemes for cervical cytology screening. This also applies to the cytology screening service within the public or private sector of medicine.

It is generally accepted as unethical to introduce a screening programme without being able to offer the necessary supportive diagnostic and treatment facilities. However, often this is not the case, and little consideration may have been given to planning for the consequences, particularly the impact on colposcopy services, of an efficient computerized call and recall scheme.

The minimum essential stages in effective cervical cancer prevention are cytological screening, diagnostic colposcopy and histological diagnosis, appropriate treatment and follow up, involving further colposcopy and cytological surveillance.

APPROXIMATION OF SERVICE REQUIREMENTS

In order to estimate the requirement for colposcopy and treatment services, there are two possible approaches. One is to determine the number of women currently screened and the existing level of diagnostic and treatment services provided to meet the demand.

An increment may then be added to account for the estimated increase in smears as a result of the introduction of the call and recall scheme. All routinely available statistics from laboratories and family practitioner committees relate to smears processed rather than women screened, and therefore the workload calculation by this method would require an ad hoc study. An alternative method is to estimate likely total demand for the services as a result of introduction of the screening programme. This second method is described here.

Calculation of demand for diagnostic colposcopy

METHOD

The demand for diagnostic colposcopy is dependent, among other things, upon the number of women screened (Table 21.1), the clinical policy for the referral of women with non-negative smears, the rate and category of non-negative smears, and referrals to the service on clinical grounds alone, regardless of a negative smear.

Table 21.1 Population screening factors	
Information required	**Source**
No. of women in the specified age groups in the population to be screened	Local age-sex register
Proportion of women who have had hysterectomy*	Estimated as 12%
Uptake rate for screening	Known or predicted
Recall interval for screening	Agreed local policy
Number of non-resident women screened	Laboratory estimates or ad hoc study

*Where previous hysterectomy has been performed in the presence of CIN, ongoing vaginal vault smears are recommended. Therefore, the estimated 12% reduction for the prevalence of hysterectomy may be excessive.

Clinical policy in relation to non-negative smears

Dyskaryosis

There is some evidence in the literature, suggesting that an initial cytological description of mild or moderate dyskaryosis may be associated with a more severe grade of cervical intraepithelial neoplasia, as shown by the final histological diagnosis, in a proportion of cases. In addition, mild dyskaryotic change may progress to a more significant grade, as may the underlying histological lesion. For these reasons, in Britain in 1987 an Intercollegiate Working Party on Cervical Cytology Screening recommended that, ideally, all women with dyskaryotic smears of any degree should be investigated by colposcopy as soon as possible. This policy has been adopted in these calculations. However, it is important to point out that more recent opinion has suggested that a repeat smear at an interval of six months is the first line of management, followed by colposcopy in the case of persistent abnormalities (see page 143).

Viral changes only

There is an association, casual or causal, between human papillomavirus infection of the cervix and squamous neoplasia. Human papillomavirus may mask underlying cervical intraepithelial neoplasia and may be associated with an increased risk of progression of the cervical intraepithelial lesion. Human papillomavirus infection also appears to be associated with an increased risk of future development of cervical intraepithelial neoplasia. It has been recommended, therefore, that the latter should be excluded in cases of human papillomavirus infection.

Other investigators have suggested that, in such cases, it may be acceptable to repeat the smear in six months, and only if cytological evidence of persistent human papillomavirus change is obtained should colposcopy be indicated. In the calculation to be described, it is assumed that colposcopy will be recommended on the initial smear showing viral changes.

Inflammatory changes only

Inflammatory changes of the cervix, and in turn in the cervical smear, may mask underlying cervical intraepithelial neoplasia. There is some reporting of a high proportion of such changes reverting to normal cytology, if the smear is repeated in three to six months. Of the remainder, approximately 50–75% may have underlying cervical intraepithelial neoplasia.

Detection of inflammatory changes in the initial smear indicates the need to identify and, where appropriate, treat any specific causal organism or agent. If non-specific inflammatory changes persist after six months, colposcopic assessment is indicated. This policy has been assumed in the calculation to be presented.

Non-negative results from population screening
Dyskaryosis

Local data, routine returns and ad hoc studies of the prevalence of dyskaryosis may be limited and complicated by a different terminology, inclusion of different degrees of dyskaryosis, and use of combinations of different numerators (smears or women) and denominators (1000 smears and 1000 women). Therefore, for the present purposes, a best working estimate of about 20 cases of dyskaryosis (any degree) per 1000 women screened will be used.

Viral changes only

Information on the prevalence of pure viral cytopathic effects as seen on smears is even more sparse and unreliable, and further complicated by the recently introduced technique, polymerase chain reaction, being used on a research basis to evaluate genital human papillomavirus infection in relatively small cohorts of the general population (see Chapter 3). The method is apparently ultrasensitive, capable of detecting a single copy of the human papillomavirus genome per 10^5 cells, either in cervical smears or in tissue biopsies. These results are currently being extended in larger studies and their proper evaluation and implications awaited.

For the moment, in routine clinical practice we must continue to rely on the simple exfoliative cytological approach to uncover subclinical human papillomavirus infection in the asymptomatic population. For a best working estimate, a figure of 10 cases per 1000 women screened will be used. It will be clear that for some populations this will be a substantial underestimate.

Inflammatory changes only

Similar problems to those relating to the prevalence of dyskaryotic changes pertain to inflammatory changes. At least one large study suggests a best working estimate of prevalence of approximately 100 cases per 1000 women screened. After a smear has been reported as showing inflammatory changes, a best estimate of 75% reverting to normal on a repeat smear after six months will be assumed and used in the subsequent calculation.

Clinical referrals

Clinical referrals because of suspicious appearances of the cervix on direct naked eye visualization, symptomatology suspicious of cervical pathology regardless of naked eye appearance (e.g. postcoital bleeding), or an overt vulval or vaginal lesion, may account for approximately 2% of the workload of a colposcopy clinic.

DERIVATION OF DEMAND FOR DIAGNOSTIC COLPOSCOPY

On the basis of the above assumptions, if 100 000 women are eligible for cervical screening, the proportion of women having had a hysterectomy is 12% (but note comment in Table 20.1); assuming the uptake for screening is 70%, and the recall interval three years; the number of non-resident women screened is 3000; then the total number of women screened per year will be:

$$\frac{[100\,000 - (12\% \times 100\,000)] \times 70\%}{3} + 3000 = 23\,533$$

The predicted number of women with dyskaryosis will be:

$$23\,533 \times 20/1000 = 471$$

The predicted number of women with viral changes only will be:

$$23\,533 \times 10/1000 = 235$$

The predicted number of women with inflammatory changes only on two consecutive smears (assuming 75% revert to normal on the second smear) will be:

$$23\,533 \times 100/1000 \times 25\% = 588$$

Therefore, the total demand for diagnostic colposcopy from screening is predicted to be:

$$471 + 235 + 588 = 1294$$

Assuming 2% of the workload is from clinical referrals, the total demand for diagnostic colposcopy will be:

$$1294 \times 102\% = 1320$$

CALCULATION OF DEMAND FOR TREATMENT

Method

The following assumption will be made: currently, the majority of women with cervical intraepithelial neoplasia receive locally destructive treatment to the transformation zone. Approximately 5% of those requiring treatment have multilevel disease involving the vagina or vulva, or extensive ectocervical or forniceal disease necessitating treatment on an inpatient basis under general anaesthesia. A further 20% of those patients that should be treated will require large excisional cone biopsy, as the lesion extends into the endocervical canal and the whole transformation zone cannot be visualized, or microinvasion/frank invasion is present or suspected.

A number of factors will influence the demand for treatment, including the number of women having diagnostic colposcopy, the proportion discharged after one colposcopic assessment, the proportion discharged after follow up colposcopy, without treatment, and the average number of attendances per woman for treatment.

PROPORTION DISCHARGED AFTER ONE COLPOSCOPIC ASSESSMENT

Approximately 50% of women with persistent inflammatory cytology can be discharged after initial colposcopy. Women with a negative first colposcopy initiated by dyskaryotic or viral changes in the smear, may have a further interval colposcopy.

PROPORTION DISCHARGED AFTER FOLLOW UP COLPOSCOPY WITHOUT TREATMENT

It will be assumed, on the basis of published literature, that 25% of women with dyskaryotic smears and 55% of women with viral changes can be discharged without treatment, after negative repeat cytology and with the precaution of follow up colposcopy.

AVERAGE NUMBER OF ATTENDANCES PER WOMAN FOR TREATMENT

The accepted success rate from one treatment by laser vaporization cone, for example, is 96%, therefore the average number of attendances per woman is 1.04.

Example calculation

Of 471 women with dyskaryotic changes, a predicted 75% will require treatment:

$$471 \times 75\% = 353$$

Of 235 women with viral changes, 45% are predicted to require treatment:

$$235 \times 45\% = 106$$

Of 588 women with inflammatory changes, 50% may require treatment:

$$588 \times 50\% = 294$$

Of 1294 referrals, some 2% or 26 women may be referred on clinical grounds. The total demand for treatment, therefore, may be:

$$353 + 106 + 294 + 26 = 779$$

Of these patients, 20% may require cone biopsy:

$$779 \times 20\% = 156$$

Also, 5% may require inpatient laser treatment:

$$779 \times 5\% = 39$$

Another 75% may require outpatient ablative therapy, such as laser vaporization cone:

$$779 \times 75\% = 584$$

If the average number of outpatient laser treatment attendances per woman is 1.04, then the required number of treatment appointments per year will be:

$$584 \times 1.04 = 607$$

CALCULATION OF DEMAND FOR FOLLOW UP COLPOSCOPY

Method

The demand for follow up colposcopy depends on the number of women receiving treatment; the average number of attendances per woman for post-treatment follow up colposcopy, and the number of women receiving follow up colposcopy without previous treatment.

AVERAGE NUMBER OF ATTENDANCES PER WOMAN FOR FOLLOW UP COLPOSCOPY AFTER TREATMENT

From an examination of local data, it will be assumed that the average attendance rate per woman for follow up colposcopy is 2.4.

Example calculation

Of 779 women to be treated, all will require colposcopic follow up after treatment. If each of these women has an average of 2.4 attendances, then the number of appointments required after treatment will be:

$$779 \times 2.4 = 1870$$

If 25% of the 471 women with dyskaryotic changes and 55% of the 235 with viral changes are to have one follow up colposcopy, then the additional requirement will be:

$$(471 \times 25\%) + (235 \times 55\%) = 118 + 129 = 247$$

Therefore, the total demand for appointments for follow up colposcopy per year will be of the order:

$$1870 + 247 = 2117$$

MEDICAL WORKLOAD IMPLICATIONS

The following are not unreasonable assumptions in trying to assess the medical requirements within the

Table 21.2   Summary of a colposcopy clinic annual workload for a population screening of 100,000 women

Activity	No.
Diagnostic colposcopy appointments	1320
Outpatient laser or other treatments	607
Inpatient laser treatments in theatre	39
Excisional cone biopsies	156
Follow up colposcopy appointments	2117

colposcopy clinic dealing with the above hypothetical overall patient numbers: the equivalent of four new patients and eight follow up patients can be seen per colposcopy table session; six outpatients can be treated per laser table session; five patients can be added to a routine gynaecology operating list for cone biopsy or local destructive treatment of cervical intraepithelial neoplasia under general anaesthesia; and all such outpatient or inpatient sessions will function for 50 working weeks per year.

On the estimates and assumptions made, the annual requirements per 100 000 women eligible for population screening would be as shown in Table 21.2.

In the example given, the requirement would be for six colposcopy table sessions per week, two laser table sessions per week, and 0.8 operating sessions per week. These figures can be compared with current provision (if any) and the additional requirements calculated. If the service also acts as a tertiary referral centre, additional capacity will be necessary. Each doctor session will require a matching nurse session, and it is likely that a clinic functioning with the doctor and nurse levels discussed above will demand the services of a full time secretary and an appointments clerk.

There is a complex relationship between non-attendance rates (which may be of the order 8% for primary diagnostic colposcopy, 10% for outpatient treatment such as laser, and 21% for follow up colposcopy), and the number of appointments required. If the non-attendance represents 'never attending', a reduction in the number of appointments would result. However, if the non-attendant eventually comes to the clinic, and the clinic is not deliberately overbooked, then an increase in the number of appointments available would be necessary. In practice, it is likely that non-attendants will be a mix of these two categories, but this is not readily quantifiable from the routinely available statistics used in the calculations presented above.

Large numbers of opportunistic smears, as opposed to 'call and recall' smears in a systematic computerized population screen, will distort the distribution of required capacity. However, assuming that smears are not unnecessarily duplicated out of phase, the total capacity should remain unchanged.

The assumptions upon which the presented model is based vary in the degree of confidence which can be attached to them, but the final result is of the right order of magnitude and is fairly robust. A major determining factor is the uptake rate in the screening programme. These assumptions are based on the available information, which is sparse. Improvements to the population screening data might soon become available, if the information from computerized 'call and recall' schemes could be analysed in relation to women rather than smears.

There will be an inevitable increase in the demand for diagnostic and treatment services, arising out of more comprehensive cervical cytology screening programmes. The data provided here should allow those concerned with service provision to plan for the capital and revenue implications of such an increase.

COLPOSCOPY CLINIC LAYOUT

Accommodation requirements at the clinic level are obviously dictated by the overall workload. For a small clinical throughput all that may be required is to have one room within an existing clinic or practice setup specially adapted to house the colposcope, with or without the facility to undertake outpatient treatment. If the latter is solely the equipment of large loop excision of the transformation zone by diathermy, for instance, then the additional space for treatment will be minimal.

On the other hand, if the technique of choice is the carbon dioxide laser, then space will be taken up by the laser console and smoke evacuation system, an essential requirement from the point of view of health and safety of staff. In addition, even in a smaller facility, it is not uncommon to find the colposcope embellished with a video television camera, with further space demanded by the television monitor. The end result is the need for a fairly commodious room.

The layout shown in Fig. 21.1 is for a purpose-built clinic sited in a large teaching hospital department of gynaecology, functioning within the public sector in the National Health Service in Britain, and offering a major proportion of the colposcopy service for a city of some 600 000 and environs, with a throughput of about 1000 new and 3500 follow up patients per year,

along with outpatient treatments thus generated.

The clinic also meets the educational needs of undergraduates and postgraduates, including short introductory courses in practical colposcopy. Currently, the favoured outpatient treatment modalities are carbon dioxide laser excision or vaporization cone and large loop excision of the transformation zone.

Description

Near the entrance, which must allow easy access for the disabled, the patient is welcomed at the reception/appointments office by the clerk. This office has a computer terminal connecting with the hospital patient administration system (PAS). This terminal also connects with the colposcopy patient records and management computer network, allowing direct transfer of basic patient biodata and appointment details between both, which is a time-saving step.

The secretary's office is nearby, with full typing facilities and the main colposcopy computer system (CPU). This office also allows temporary storage of active standard hardcopy hospital case records, for current patients.

Proceeding through the clinic, there is the patient waiting area, with comfortable seating, a hot drinks dispenser and piped music. Adequate toilet facilities are essential, which must also cater for males and the disabled.

A small technical maintenance laboratory is provided, allowing a safe area for the servicing of laser equipment by the hospital medical physics department staff. For this reason, this room has an appropriate illuminated laser sign at the entrance. The ability to conduct a minimal level of in-house laser maintenance is essential for the smooth running of the treatment sessions.

A small staff rest room is provided, with a seminar room adjacent to it, reflecting the teaching role of the clinic. This latter room has slide projection facilities and video playback equipment, with a monitor that can also be connected via a network of video cables to any of the video cameras in the four colposcopy examination/treatment rooms.

Finally, a computer terminal as part of the patient records and management system is also located here, both as a work terminal and as a demonstration point during the short practical courses for postgraduates.

The clinical area is designed so that four doctor table sessions can be run simultaneously. There are four colposcopy rooms, with integral patient changing cubicle. Histories are taken at a desk with a computer terminal consisting of a visual display unit and keyboard linked via a network to the CPU in the secretary's office. Patient details are entered 'real time'. All four rooms are kitted for diagnostic colposcopy and biopsy, but two are larger to accommodate the additional equipment for laser surgery.

Each room has a video television option, with the monitor in sight of the patient. This is a useful arrangement for explaining findings and giving an indication of what the treatment involves. Most

women are appreciative of this facility, which has been included primarily as a teaching aid both for colposcopists in training and for the nursing staff.

These examination rooms are paired so as to be served by a small utility room where trolleys are set up, waste disposal units are available and CSSD packs etc. stored. At a central point of access in the clinical area there is a resuscitation trolley, for the

Fig. 21.1 Layout for a large dedicated colposcopy facility, fulfilling diagnostic, treatment and teaching roles. The maintenance room is designated for in-house maintenance of carbon dioxide lasers. Other aspects of the layout are self-explanatory.

unlikely event of profound vasovagal or other collapse in a patient receiving attention in the clinic. Minor vasovagal episodes are not uncommon in a busy clinic, after punch biopsy or even apparently straightforward diagnostic colposcopy.

22. Epilogue

EVOLVING TECHNOLOGY

Histopathology

The histological appearances covered in earlier chapters are based on routinely processed material stained with haematoxylin and eosin. These basic techniques have long been the mainstay of histological diagnosis and are likely to remain so for the foreseeable future. Their use, however, is based on the assumption that the morphological features that are capable of analysis by these methods allow some prediction of the biological potential of the tissue under study. In many areas of histopathology this assumption may be acceptable for practical purposes, but its applicability to some areas of lower genital tract pathology is questionable. This is particularly the case for the prediction of the malignant potential of cervical intraepithelial neoplasia, but is also true for glandular abnormalities and microinvasive carcinoma. There is hope that a reappraisal of the histological grading system for squamous intraepithelial lesions combined with a careful redefining of diagnostic criteria may go some way towards improving the predictive value of conventional histology for this condition. Even so, the accuracy of this method of diagnosis is still likely to fall far short of the ideal that should be attained. Attention is therefore being turned to the use of alternative methods, in an attempt to assess the neoplastic and malignant potential of tissues.

Nucleic acid analyses, using nucleic acid probes, are capable of identifying the sequences which make up a segment of a gene. The gene in question may be of any type, those currently of most interest being of viral origin, oncogenes and antioncogenes. A variety of techniques are available for applying the nucleic acid probes to the tissue: solid-support hybridization assays include dot/blot/slot hybridization and their variants, Southern and Northern hybridization. These methods involve digestion of tissue and therefore destruction of its architecture. In situ hybridization allows the nucleic acid probe to be applied to a histological section, so that the distribution of the genomic sequences can be determined. These techniques also allow an attempt at quantitation to be made. An amplification procedure, the polymerase chain reaction (PCR), amplifies specific DNA sequences and may be used when the gene to be detected is only present in single copies per cell, or when the amount of sample DNA to be analysed is very small.

At present, the practical applications of these DNA techniques, used either individually or in combination, in cervical pathology include the identification of human papillomavirus and its subtypes within the epithelium, and the recognition and quantitation of various oncogenes. It is expected that many new applications will emerge in the future.

Immunocytochemistry depends upon a reaction in which antibodies (often monoclonal but sometimes polyclonal) raised against selected antigenic determinants bind to that antigen. The site of binding is indicated by a colour change (a peroxidase: antiperoxidase reaction is usually employed, resulting in a brown colour), so that the distribution of the antigen in the tissue can be determined. The reaction is also often considered to be capable of some degree of quantitation. A very wide variety of antigens can be identified with immunocytochemistry such as intermediate filaments (cytokeratins, desmin, vimentin etc.), growth factor receptors and oncogene protein products.

Finally, mention must be made of flow cytometry, the main application of which has been in cell ploidy analysis. The analysis is carried out on disaggregated tissue and so the origin of the nuclei measured is not always certain. Slide-based image processing technology may well replace flow cytometric instruments for DNA ploidy analysis, because of the increased ability of the operator to control and monitor the process, including selection of the cells for measurement. Flow cytometry may also be used for measuring monoclonal antibody uptake of cells.

This account lists only some of the new techniques which are currently being investigated. The majority of the information available is too preliminary to justify the inclusion of any of these methods in the diagnostic or prognostic evaluation of a particular patient's lesion, and much more investigation is required to ascertain which markers, genetic and otherwise, will be useful in this clinical field. Because these techniques are able to identify an ever increasing variety of cellular characteristics, which are quite distinct from those recognized by conventional methods, it is hoped that eventually a marker or, more probably, a series of markers, such as nucleic acid sequences or cell surface receptors, will be identified which will allow an accurate assessment of neoplastic state and malignant potential.

Cytology

The DNA hybridization and immunocytochemistry techniques outlined above have already led to great advances in cytology, both in routine diagnosis and research, although at the moment they are used to the greatest benefit in non-gynaecological areas. Many of these techniques are at least as applicable to cytology as to histopathology, and their use results in an even greater blurring of the artificial disinction between the disciplines.

Automated screening offers the greatest potential for radical change in gynaecological cytology. However, despite the immense sums that have been spent over many years of development, the cell counter and flow cytometry methods still have not achieved acceptable levels of reliability or cost effectiveness for widespread use in routine laboratories. Currently, the greatest promise for automated screening lies with imaging techniques. Early attempts were disappointing, but the most recent advances in computer technology, with the emergence of neural network systems, have led to the development of small, mobile prototype systems that could be readily sited in all cytology departments, even the smallest, at a cost of only a few pounds per smear examined.

Neurocomputer imaging systems carry many advantages. The cervical smear is taken and prepared in the standard way, without the need for the special processing that other experimental automated systems have required. The computer automatically analyses a large number of images taken from the slide, and the slide itself is then available for subsequent review by conventional light microscopy, thus eliminating the need for immediate recall of the patient. Furthermore, the images of cells analysed by the computer are presented to the observer in exactly the same way as they appear in the cervical smear, so that minimal additional training is necessary.

The ever increasing problems of providing and maintaining adequate numbers of trained staff in cytology departments make the idea of developing automated screening systems that are able to identify safely the majority of truly negative cervical smears, more attractive than ever. The neural network automatic computerized imaging system is the most exciting development to date, and has the potential to achieve this aim.

GUIDELINES FOR TRAINING IN COLPOSCOPY

Most authorities accept that colposcopy training can be broken down into two categories, basic and advanced colposcopy, but there is still some disagreement as to when a colposcopist passes from one grade to the next.

Basic colposcopy implies an understanding of the principles of colposcopy and problems which the colposcopist will be asked to assess. It also implies a knowledge of various treatment options which are available if treatment proves necessary. Ideally, all trainee gynaecologists should receive training in basic colposcopy, in the same way that they are trained in ultrasound scanning, laparoscopy, etc. Many of them will never have to use it, but at least they have knowledge of it and of its potential.

This form of training will be of an ongoing nature and usually taught on a one-to-one basis. On the other hand, throughout the world there are many specialist gynaecologists with no knowledge of colposcopy, who wish to learn about it. The subject cannot be learnt from a book, and the recommended introduction to colposcopy is to attend a two-day theoretical course of instruction, followed by a course of practical work with a tutor.

Both may be extremely difficult in some parts of the world, but nevertheless colposcopy should not be practised unless there has' been an opportunity to spend some time with an experienced colposcopist. The aim of basic colposcopy is to demonstrate what the colposcopist looks at and what should be done once the diagnosis has been made. The basic colposcopist should be very wary of relying on destructive methods of treatment, in case unsuspected invasive carcinoma is missed, and should therefore use colposcopy as a guide to planning excisional methods of treatment.

On the other hand, advanced colposcopy cannot be taught simply, quickly or easily. It requires many months of intensive training in a unit which receives many hundreds or even thousands of cases per year. This will allow the student not only to recognize the basic colposcopic patterns, but also to become skilled in the management of lower genital tract premalignancy. The advanced colposcopist also needs to recognize lesions which are not intraepithelial neoplasia, such as immature metaplasia, congenital transformation zone, human papillomavirus infection, changes due to simple atrophy, and changes due to radiotherapy.

All of these can confuse even the most experienced colposcopist, and it is important that lesions are recognized for what they are, rather than committing a patient to a course of surgical treatment which may turn out to be totally unnecessary.

Unfortunately, such training is time consuming and may not be widely available; therefore, the limitations of basic colposcopy need to be clearly defined so that a colposcopist with no more than basic training is not tempted to embark on treatment regimens which are beyond his or her capabilities.

At whatever level colposcopy is to be practised, some knowledge of cytology and histopathology is essential, together with a good working relationship between those specializing in the three disciplines.

As regards the question of who should be trained in colposcopy, traditionally, only gynaecologists have practised it, but clinical gynaecological training is not mandatory. Pathologists interested in the cervix can make excellent colposcopists. In some parts of the world, nurses have been trained to perform basic colposcopy, particularly in countries where there are not enough doctors, or the patients cannot afford the fee of a medically trained colposcopist. There is no reason why a nurse should not be trained in basic colposcopy, and this can be compared to the question: 'who should deliver babies, midwives or obstetricians?' Throughout the world, midwives carry a great responsibility, but only after a period of very intensive training.

Similarly, in Britain, some colposcopists are general practitioners with no specialist training in gynaecology, but who nevertheless have been trained in the rudiments of colposcopy and do an excellent job: not only does this training provide colposcopists, but it also allows highly trained gynaecologists to be free for other clinical duties.

Colposcopy cannot be learnt from a book or by attending a two-day course. It is the responsibility of colposcopy societies in different countries to provide training in their own territories. Members of each national society should have the opportunity to meet on an annual basis and discuss current problems and techniques. The formation of the International Federation of Cervical Pathology and Colposcopy in 1972 made it possible to meet at an international level every third year. Meetings such as these teach us that training is never complete, and new techniques, new drugs and new principles evolve year after year.

Index

Numbers given in bold are figures; tables have the prefix 'tab(s)' CIN is entered under Intraepithelial neoplasia (CIN)